# Smoke Screens:
# The Truth About Tobacco

ISBN number: 978 1 4092 4670 1

A CIP catalogue record for this book is available from the British Library

Visit www.smokescreens.org to contact the author or for more information on *Smoke Screens: The Truth About Tobacco* including regular articles and a forum.

Published in collaboration with Lulu
3101 Hillsborough Street
Raleigh, NC, 27607
USA.
Printed in the USA

*With thanks to:*

*Everyone who has offered support to this book being written and completed*

*Special Acknowledgements:*

*Linda Stewart, for her contributions to Chapter 6 with an article originally published as "The Case Against Smoking Bans" for N.Y.C. C.L.A.S.H.*

*Lauren Colby, for his continued support and contributions to this entire book*

*Dr Ian Dunbar, for the suggestions, contributions and support*

*Chris Snowdon, for the constructive criticism*

*Michael McFadden for his selfless help*

# Contents

# Foreword

It is a common student experience to be taught things one knows deep down are just not true.

In the 1950s, when Professor Richard Doll published his research linking smoking and lung cancer, I was a medical student. Everyone in the class scoffed. If smoking caused lung cancer why did so many smokers die of old age? Since those early days I have viewed each new statistical revelation with a pinch of salt.

In this conscientious, painstaking and scholarly review of the literature, Richard White has validated my scepticism. The book is encyclopaedic in its content. Among the many topics embraced is 'detection bias' whereby the notion that smoking causes cancer is now so ingrained that the possibility of lung cancer when doctors examine non-smokers is overlooked; they are not expecting to find cancer and so do not investigate appropriately. Researchers still do not know precisely how, or indeed whether, smoking causes cancer or any of the other diseases attributed to it; they have struggled with weird and wonderful experiments to try and produce tumours in laboratory animals and failed dismally. The chemicals in tobacco smoke are similar to those in traffic fumes, except that in traffic fumes the concentration is much higher; cigarette smoke is therefore less toxic than the air we ordinarily breathe. In the final analysis, all that researchers have accomplished is to produce tenuous statistical links that they regard as 'significant'. Examples of the disordered thought that has lain behind these tenuous links are also outlined.

Often forgotten is the fact that tobacco itself warns of its hazards. All smokers can recall that first puff that made them cough and splutter; indeed it made some vomit. The first lesson tobacco teaches is to take care when inhaling. Like all such experiences it is a question of moderation. Smoke too much for too long and the result is a smoker's cough. But an excess of abstinence is equally hazardous; the fanaticism of the anti-smoking lobby graphically illustrates this.

The medical profession possesses more knowledge than one individual can master in a lifetime of learning. Professional organisation has evolved to cope by a division of labour into researchers, consultants and general practitioners. Researchers and consultants specialise in small areas of medical knowledge, studying in depth. General practitioners, on the other hand, acquire a more general knowledge of medicine, studying in breadth. Had they been better organised, researchers, consultants and general practitioners, working together as a team, could have made medical knowledge available to society both in depth and in perspective.

Unfortunately, researchers and consultants see themselves as superior and take a disparaging view of general clinical practice. In the National Health Service they routinely keep family doctors waiting weeks, even months, for a second opinion. But good family doctors really want that opinion by tomorrow. This is because they realise that their patients are anxious to know the result and seek to minimise that anxiety.

The General Medical Council's own rules regard 'disparagement' as 'professional misconduct'. But Council has routinely turned a blind eye so that professional misconduct has become institutionalised. The result is that the medical profession has lost all sense of proportion; researchers and consultants have no idea of the problems presenting in the family doctor's consulting room from the world at large.

If one looks more closely at those problems, one finds that some 75% of cases are the physical symptoms of anxiety such as headaches, indigestion, diarrhoea, palpitations and general aches and pains. These symptoms mimic more serious physical illness and it is the clinical judgement of the family doctor that determines whether indigestion is caused by anxiety or cancer of the stomach, for example. About 24% of cases are minor infections such as coughs and sore throats. Serious physical illnesses of the kind described in medical text books, such as pneumonia, cancer and heart disease are very rare. Modern medical science is in fact totally ignorant of the causes and cures of most of the illness in the community. Over the years, ever more resources have been devoted to studying rarer and rarer conditions. But propaganda in the media would have people believe that medical science is on the brink of knowing it all.

There are two scientific methods: one is appropriate for studying inanimate objects like tobacco; the other is appropriate for studying animate objects such as people. The difference between them is that the study of inanimate objects excludes all reference to non-material or metaphysical states such as the mind. But to be scientific, all the variables affecting any given situation must be considered. Much of the confusion surrounding research into the effects of tobacco arises from the fact that a scientific method appropriate for studying inanimate objects such as tobacco has been deployed to study the effects of tobacco on animate objects such as people.

In effect, researchers have been overlooking the fact that there are two realities in the everyday lives of people: there is the shared objective reality of the world around us and there is the personal subjective reality of our own thoughts and feelings. However, subjective reality is not actually all in the mind. It is modulated by powerful hormones such as adrenaline, which has wide-ranging effects on both the mind and the body. For example, adrenaline not only causes the subjective reality of apprehension and anxiety which are difficult to measure, it also affects objective reality by raising pulse rate and blood pressure which are easy to measure.

For most people, most of the time, subjective reality is preoccupied by hopes, fears, jealousies, grievances, and suchlike. Only rarely does it cause the physical symptoms for which a family doctor is consulted. These hopes and fears merely distract people and can be referred to as the chattering apes of consciousness.

Numerous studies have shown that plasma b-endorphin concentrations (natural opiates in the body) increase in a dose-related manner after administration of nicotine. This means that nicotine has a sedative effect. But this effect is very mild and in no way compares to the sedative effect of ingested opiates. It is therefore easily overlooked. But the reason why people smoke is to obtain this mild sedative effect.

The more insecure people are, the more they will smoke. But the more insecure people are the greater the amount of adrenaline that will be produced. The greater the amount of adrenaline produced the higher the blood pressure and pulse rate are likely to be raised, and the greater the chances of suffering a stroke. Chronic insecurity is therefore likely to ultimately result in heart disease and strokes. This is illustrated by the fact that while poorer people tend to smoke heavily, single parents in particular, their lives are more fraught; they are therefore more likely to die younger anyway.

In the final analysis, heart disease, strokes and smoking all have a common causative denominator in insecurity. It is this common denominator that creates the illusion of a significant statistical link.

# Foreword

Ian Dunbar M.B.Ch.B

# Introduction: Where It All Began

Until the 1950s almost nobody would have suggested smoking was harmful, let alone deadly. Doctors even recommended smoking; my own grandmother's doctor told her to smoke during her pregnancy in order to eat less. There are videos on Youtube of old cigarette advertisements in which doctors recommend smoking – one Camel advert has doctors saying they favour that particular brand over others.[1] Smoking was not only socially acceptable, it was the norm; almost everybody smoked. One look at classical Hollywood will show just how prominent smoking was at the time. Moreover, smoking was seen as classy and elegant – who can forget the classic picture of Audrey Hepburn with her cigarette holder? Even today smoking is widely used in films and art to symbolise anything from a phallic symbol to independence. An example of this is the film *Fight Club*, in which a cigarette was used to symbolise masculinity. Until more recent times, it was commonplace in Europe for people to keep spare cigarettes and an ashtray to offer their guests upon arrival in their home. Smoking was so entrenched within society that when the idea that it could be harmful first came to light most doctors, and indeed civilians, refuted the idea as preposterous.

The very first study showing that smoking was linked to lung cancer was conducted in 1912 by Dr. Isaac Adler who used a monograph to demonstrate the link. As early as 1928 there were studies in Germany also purporting to demonstrate a link, although the first formal statistical evidence was in 1929 by Fritz Lickint of Dresden. This study was far from conclusive though, as the link was simply 'discovered' because men smoked more than women and had higher incidence of lung cancer than women. The other German studies will be looked at in the sub-chapter 'The Nazi Discovery of Smoking and Cancer'.

Despite these earlier attempts to demonise tobacco, the public perception of smoking did change. The pinnacle study to the current anti-smoking movement was conducted by Sir Richard Doll.

Doll was, and despite his passing still remains, one of the most prominent figures in the anti-smoking movement. After the publication of his first study in 1950 he was very active in speaking out against smoking. Cancer Research UK, speaking of this study, state on their website "This British Doctors Study has provided

---

[1] http://www. youtube.com/watch?v=gCMzjJjuxQI

much of our current knowledge about the dangers of smoking."[2] On the fiftieth anniversary, June 2004, Doll released the follow up, a fifty-year epidemiological study. Research shows that much of today's figures and statistics on the hazards of smoking come from this study; it is considered the Holy Grail of smoking studies and, as far as the Tobacco Control movement is concerned, it has not yet been surpassed. In looking at the study in detail later on, the reader will probably have to question the validity of such figures and subsequent claims.

That study prompted a lot of change: an ever increasing number of studies began to emerge showing a correlation between smoking and lung cancer, and then studies that linked smoking with emphysema and heart disease. Nowadays, there is barely a week that goes by without another anti-smoking revelation, to the point where we are now told smoking can cause a range of cancers including bowel, pancreatic and bladder, as well as impotence, aging of the skin, acne and even blindness! We are also continually told that second-hand smoke is responsible for thousands of deaths each and every year.

What started off as somewhat feasible – that inhaling smoke into the lungs could cause lung cancer – is now looking hugely different: never before has there been such an attack on any substance (except perhaps alcohol in the 1920s), despite well known and well documented dangers of countless chemicals in our everyday purchases. No other product of substance has received such hounding, and it seems the evidence, whilst getting more and more plentiful, is becoming more and more far fetched. In 2007 the United Kingdom implemented a blanket smoking ban, meaning the legal activity is now prohibited in any enclosed area including pubs, clubs, and even open-air railway platforms.

The first thing most people ask is 'how does banning smoking benefit the government?' A good question and the answer is simultaneously somewhat obvious and surprising: money. Anti-smoking groups, such as Action on Smoking and Health (ASH) (UK), receive funding for their work, whilst most pro-smoking groups, such as Fight Ordinances and Restrictions to Control and Eliminate Smoking (FORCES), receive no such funding. Furthermore, the funding to ASH and other such groups comes, in

[2]http://info.cancerresearchuk.org/healthyliving/smokingandtobacco/howdoweknow/

part, from the Department of Health. Freedom Organisation for the Right To Enjoy Smoking Tobacco (FOREST), on the other hand, is one of the few, if not the only, pro-smoking group to receive funding and this comes from the tobacco industry itself. The government has, therefore, aligned itself with one side instead of remaining neutral.

The aforementioned study by Doll was funded by the Medical Research Council, Cancer Research UK and the British Heart Foundation,[3] and Cancer Research's "Smoke is Poison" campaign was funded by the Department of Health.[4] Suing Big Tobacco was, at one time, hugely rewarding – financially speaking. The anti-smoking campaign allows government members to increase the size and power of their agencies and further their careers, whilst allowing those outside the government increased funding for their research projects. Some people may be thinking 'but they put a lot of money into anti-smoking adverts'. In truth, the anti-smoking adverts and campaigns are funded by the excessive tax on cigarettes so that it is smokers themselves who are paying for the adverts. Furthermore, there are now countless products designed to help people stop smoking, such as patches and gum (including a different type of gum for every each type of cigarette) as well as in-person individual support and treatment. Smoking cessation lines many pockets with a lot of money.

What is widely overlooked, ignored, or just not known is that a very definite health establishment exists, to which organisations like the National Health Service (NHS) and Cancer Research UK belong. Within this health establishment are the researchers and scientists who depend upon funding for their research. There is now a bandwagon, so to speak; any anti-smoking study is guaranteed to receive grants, and guaranteed to get exposure. Thus, the bigger picture begins to emerge and we can see that scientists and researchers are almost forced to churn out anti-smoking studies, regardless of how bogus they are. As a matter of fact, there is a large, and increasing, body of evidence showing tobacco smoke helps prevent Parkinson's and Alzheimer's, as well as relieving symptoms of Tourette's syndrome; unfortunately one has

---

[3]http://info.cancerresearchuk.org/news/archive/pressreleases/2004/june/38863

[4] http://info.cancerresearchuk.org/healthyliving/smokeispoison/?a=5441

to dig around a bit before finding the studies, reinforcing the above point, but we will get to them in chapter thirteen.

Some people believe that tobacco has been scrutinised as a cover-up because the establishment still has no answer to what causes cancer. The idea is certainly conceivable, even probable. As a matter of fact, in 1952 the American Cancer Society (ACS) was frustrated that there was no known cure for cancer, or even a known cause of it, and accused smoking so as to appear to the public they were onto something. In the same year, the ACS conducted a study in which volunteers were used under the assumption they would be researching whether smoking was related to lung cancer or not, but in actual fact they were setting out to prove smoking did cause lung cancer. Dr Leroy E. Burney, Surgeon General at the time, supported the ACS' claim that smoking causes lung cancer, allowing further exposure for the claim, saying "Unless the use of tobacco can be made safe, the individual person's risk of lung cancer can best be reduced by the elimination of smoking."[5]

Another small but relevant point to raise is just what a smoking ban potentially means – and certainly what people stopping smoking means. While the government, NHS and anti-smoking groups are quick to inform people that smokers cost the NHS between £1.5 and £2.7 billion a year in treatment, what they are not so quick to tell people is that smokers pay *into* society over £9 billion annually through cigarette tax. It does not require a mathematician to work out that no government is going to willingly lose that amount of money, and as such the more the smoking rates decrease, the more other taxes will have to increase. Will people be so pleased if the ban is working and there are fewer smokers around so other taxes have to rise? I, for one, doubt it.

Elaborating on the above point, it is important to keep in mind that when we are told smokers cost the NHS £1.5 billion annually, what that means is that any smoker needing treatment is categorised as having a smoking-related illness – whether the doctor believes it was smoking-related or not. In fact, the smoking-related illness figures comprise everyone *thought* to be ill from smoke, including any smoker, regardless of the illness, any non-smoker

---

[5] http://legacy.library.ucsf.edu/tid/cmq36b00/pdf

who lives with a smoker and anyone claiming to be exposed to second-hand smoke.[6]

Furthermore, 'smoking-related disease' is an incredibly misleading term as there is not a single illness or ailment that affects only smokers, and as such it cannot be a 'smoking-related disease'; such a term would relate to something that only afflicts smokers, or at least, an ailment which was caused solely by the act of smoking. There is no way of telling whether a smoker would have contracted the same illness if he or she did not smoke, and consequently the statistics are misleading. Given that statistics are the main body of research it is imperative to keep that point in mind. It is one thing to say that 50% of smokers die of smoking-related diseases, but that is an irrelevant point – official statistics also say that smoking is "the cause of more than a quarter (29%) of all deaths from cancer and has killed an estimated six million people over the last 50 years."[7] This means, of course, that 71% of cancer deaths are *not* from smoking, yet it appears to be the main focus of research. Moreover, the word "estimated" is a subtle way of saying unproven, thus allowing those who announce the figures an ability to create any number they desire.

Let us have one last look at the official statistics from Cancer Research: "Around one in four British adults currently smoke. Men are still more likely to smoke than women (27% and 25% respectively)."[8] However, the official census shows that, in 2001, there were 58.8 million people living in Britain, of which 11.9 million were under sixteen, leaving 46.9 million over sixteen. For argument's sake, we will consider those aged 16 or over as adults and, again for argument's sake, we will work under the assumption that 50% are male and 50% female. This means 23.45 million are men and 23.45 million are female. 27% of 23.45 is 6,331,500 and 25% is 5,862,500. Combining these totals leaves us with 12,194,000 smokers in the UK, or 26% of the population.

Using the above statistics, 26% of the adult population smoke, which is 12.19 million, and apparently 50% of smokers die

---

[6] Levy, R; Marimont, R (1998) *Lies, Damn Lies & 400,000 Smoking-Related Deaths*

[7] http://info.cancerresearchuk.org/cancerstats/causes/lifestyle/tobacco/

[8] Ibid

from cancer, a total of six million. If this is the case, how is it that only six million people in the UK have died from tobacco in the last fifty years, especially as the rates of smokers have declined in the same space of time?[9] Clearly, something is amiss. Of course, those are just statistics from Cancer Research; in 1990 Richard Peto – a researcher who worked with Doll – claimed that cigarette smoking was responsible for 20% of deaths in the Western world. The problem is that either figures are too low, showing that, with the amount of people who do smoke or have smoked, there is statistically no risk to the habit, or that they are too high, showing nothing but sheer manipulation and propaganda. Furthermore, one would expect the figures to be at least vaguely similar, yet they are not.

Sadly, because conventional wisdom states that smoking is harmful and carries a strong risk that it will cause cancer, people passively accept this. However, not only is there plenty of evidence that this conventional wisdom is wrong, but history itself shows that conventional wisdom is often incorrect. In the first instance, doctors used to advise smoking – so they were either wrong then or now. Additionally, alcohol was prohibited and then allowed again. Let us also not forget that, before the 1900s, it was a commonly held belief, still used jokingly today, that masturbation causes blindness. People readily accepted this and truly believed masturbation was a high risk activity, yet we now know that it is not. However, no person in their right mind, doctors or other professionals especially, would have said otherwise because if their words influenced someone to go ahead and masturbate and the person coincidentally went blind, masturbation and the doctor would have been blamed. It was also believed, and stated by experts, that marijuana would turn people into sex-crazed murderous maniacs. Some people may also remember how, in the 1970s and 1980s, parents were instructed to put their babies to sleep face down, which resulted in a huge increase in the number of cot deaths.

These examples show that conventional wisdom can be incorrect and lead people in the wrong direction. The sad truth is that because the mantra of smoking being harmful has been repeated so many times people now just accept it without question

---

[9] Ibid

or research. However, misinformation or a lie told over and over is still wrong; never will mere repetition make something true.

One argument I hear often from anti-smokers, when they are told of the evidence that smoking is not as harmful as we are told, is that it is propaganda from the tobacco industry or those receiving funding from them, such as FORCES. However, FORCES, and most other freedom of choice groups, receive no funding from any organisation. Furthermore, most of the evidence used by those groups is actually the same studies that are used to show smoking is harmful, they just point out the bias present in the studies, or intentionally missed factors that had skewed the results, and so forth. In other words, the very studies used to show smoking is harmful have been, or can be, reviewed to show that, actually, they do no such thing. Perhaps the most relevant quote is from Winston Churchill when he said: "a lie gets halfway around the world before the truth gets a chance to put its pants on".

Another odd mantra that is oft spoken by anti-smokers is that tobacco is the only product in the world that, when used as it is intended, kills its users. It is amazing that they had the temerity to think this up, and even more amazing that people repeat it with conviction. Apparently, none of these people think of vehicle accidents where a car tyre blows out, or people who eat too much food thus becoming obese and dying (after all, they consumed the food the way it was meant to be consumed: eating it), or drinking too much alcohol, or, most surprisingly, illegal drugs.

This book will be looking objectively at studies that have been used to prove smoking is harmful. It will also be looking at what other scientists really think of the existing anti-smoking studies. This book will not be choosing select studies in an attempt to disprove the existing mantra that smoking can cause death, as that would be a pointless and childish exercise akin to one person saying 'yes it does' and another saying 'no it doesn't'. Instead, it will be focusing on studies that are widely used as evidence for smoking being harmful to see if those conclusions are really true, as well as reviewing other bodies of work for a well-rounded and neutral standpoint on smoking to see whether or not smoking has an effect on the body that warrants any alarm.

Before continuing, it is important to include a disclaimer: I do not, nor have ever, worked for, or received money from, tobacco or medical* companies or other bodies on behalf of the tobacco or medical industries. I do not, nor have ever, owned shares or stocks in any tobacco or medical company. The following work was not conducted under any premise or promise of receiving money in the future from tobacco or medical companies, nor is it intended as advocacy of smoking. The book is an independent and neutral analysis of various factors in the smoking controversy.

I have included citations of all my references and where possible I have cited links to web pages. In most instances the web pages are there for the reader's convenience as they contain the original articles in their entirety and so save hunting libraries for the documents. In the instances where the original documents are not on the web page they are either scientific articles or contain information from relevant documents – again, I have included them to save those who want to check the references from spending time locating the original articles or documents.

* 'Medical' includes pharmaceutical or any other related companies

# Chapter 1: The Black Lung Myth

A common idea, amongst smokers and non-smokers alike, is that smoking causes tar deposits in the lungs. It is believed these tar deposits turn the lungs black and cause cancer.[10] Cancer Research UK says of tar that it is "a sticky black residue made up of thousands of chemicals that stays in the smoker's lungs and causes cancer." However, it does not take much logical thought and science to realise this not only *is not* true, but *cannot* be true. The idea that smoking causes black lungs is no more than a myth, and the evidence for this is plentiful.

Possibly the first thing people say on the subject is that they have seen pictures of a smoker's blackened lung and a non-smoker's pink lung. While it may be true that the blackened lung was that of a smoker and the pink lung that of a non-smoker, that is not the end of the story; the pictures are invariably of a smoker's cancerous lung and a healthy non-smoker's lung, and we now know that cancerous organs often turn black. A report in MNDaily[11] on a cancer exhibition called *Cancer and the Human Body* explained that, as part of the event, a black, oversized lung was shown next to a normal healthy lung to show the effects of lung cancer. What this serves to show is that lung cancer will usually turn the organ black.

A few years ago channel four ran a series of programmes showing autopsies conducted live by Dr Von Hagens, and one episode was on cancer. The woman having the autopsy performed was ravaged with cancer and it was very obvious which organs were cancerous by their colour: they were all black. Of course, not all cancerous organs are black, and indeed some are dyed for the purpose of education or scare-mongering.

Going back to the pictures of the two lungs, the fact that the smoker's lung is always cancerous and the non-smoker's lung always healthy means they are incomparable. If a smoker's lung was compared with a non-smoker's lung and neither had cancer then they would both look identical, and the same is true for a smoker's and non-smoker's lung with cancer. Furthermore, the photographs are invariably of the outside of the lung and not the inside.

---

[10] http://www.cnn.com/HEALTH/9610/17/nfm/smoking.gun/index.html

[11] http://www.mndaily.com/2008/02/25/cancer-exhibit-educates-and-entertains-local-museum

Cigarette smoke never reaches the outside of the lung and subsequently would have no chance to turn it black.

The original run of such photographs was pulled in 1969 as it was discovered that the lungs portrayed as smokers were, in fact, those of coal miners whose lungs had turned black from years of exposure to the soot and carbon.[12] If smoking really was responsible for blackening the lungs, no such trickery would have been necessary.

In 1964 the U.S. Tobacco Research Council conducted a study of 3,000 lungs taken at autopsy for atypical metaplasia. The researchers found no difference between smokers and non-smokers. Also in 1964, in Germany, a study consisting of 26,000 autopsy records found that there was no significant relationship between smoking and lung cancer.

Today, even those conducting autopsies admit that looking at lungs alone is not a way to tell if the deceased smoked. Wray Kephart is a man who used to work in hospitals performing autopsies, usually on the behalf of insurance companies. Writing online, Kephart claims to have performed around 1560 autopsies and he says it is normally impossible to tell whether the deceased was a smoker or not from autopsy. This was confirmed by Dr Jan Zeldenrust, a Dutch pathologist for the Government of Holland from 1951-1984. In a television interview in the 1980s he stated:

> I could never see on a pair of lungs if they belonged to a smoker or non-smoker. I can see clearly the difference between sick and healthy lungs. The only black lungs I've seen are from peat-workers and coal miners, never from smokers.[13]

Further confirmation came recently when I was able to speak to a Canadian Licensed Practical Nurse (LPN) named Adam Highberg. The discussion was mainly about oral cancers but he also spoke briefly about smokers' lungs, saying:

---

[12] http://isaac.idkcomp.com/EDTORIAL/TAR.HTM

[13] Translated from Dutch. The interview was published in a local Dutch newspaper *Limburgs Dagblad*. An online transcription in the original language can be seen at: http://www.nujij.nl/rokers-sterven-zeven-jaar-eerder-tien-feiten.3184158.lynkx

I have seen diseased lungs before, and sometimes in the case of smokers, but not always. These are normally found in people who live and work in unhealthy environments for extended periods of time. You know, the guy who works in a fibreglass plant but never wears a mask. Because of this, it would be almost impossible to say that black lungs are solely that of smoking; I believe that it is far more likely an environment issue.

The lungs are always clear unless the deceased had lung cancer or heavy exposure to pollution, such as that from living in a large city or an occupation like coal mining.

Living in a city, or any area with a significant amount of pollution, is one factor that many people are unaware of or choose to ignore when it comes to the state of the lungs. Anyone who lives in, or visits, such a place will be aware of the black that they either cough up or produce when blowing their nose, and it is this same produce that can be seen in X-rays on the lungs. The produce in question is elemental carbon, which will indeed stick to the lungs and living in a built-up area for a long time can turn the inside of the lungs somewhat black.

A little test for those with curiosity, or who just want to see for themselves, is to simply ask someone who lives in a city, and has done for a long time, to go for an X-ray and see how their lungs look. Similarly, ask a long-term smoker, not from a city, to go for the same X-ray and compare the results. With the exception of extreme cases, such as those who smoke over three packs (sixty cigarettes) a day, doctors are unable to tell if someone smokes just by looking at their lungs.

Of course, there are always individual exceptions: not all cancerous organs are black, and not all city-living folk will have black lungs. It is important to stress also that those in highly polluted areas do not have jet black lungs like fear-mongering science pictures purport, but will have black particle staining.

Another common misconception is that cigarettes contain tar – they do not; at least, not the type of tar that is used on roads as many people now believe. As stated at the start of this chapter, the general belief is the tar from cigarettes deposits in the lungs and causes cancer. This simply is not the case. If, indeed, cigarettes caused tar to be deposited in the lungs of smokers then each and every one would die of asphyxiation long before they ever got the chance to get cancer. Researchers would also be able to simply put tar in the lungs of animals and wait for the cancer to develop, yet this has never been the case. Tar is a very thick substance and it can kill people very easily. In the days when Christianity was illegal, one of the methods of killing the martyrs was by having their bodies dipped in tar. The tar blocked up their pores and prevented their skin being able to breathe, thus killing them. Clearly, there is no way someone could live with much tar in their lungs. Furthermore, if there was tar present in cigarettes it would not only be in the lungs, but also in the mouth and throat as well as on teeth and fingers, and smokers would cough up chunks of black tar. This has never happened. Let us take a look at the facts:

In America, full-strength cigarettes contain 20 mg of 'tar'. The lung capacity of an average adult human is about six litres, or 6,000 cubic centimetres.[14] At room temperature, one cubic centimetre (one ml) of water weighs about one gram. However, tar is an oily substance that floats on water, so one millilitre weighs less than a gram. The exact density of tar depends on its composition, but tar is usually a mixture of many different oily chemicals and at its densest one gram occupies about 1.25 ml of volume. At 20 mg (0.025 ml) of 'tar' per cigarette, it would take at least 50 cigarettes, or two and a half packs, to yield one gram of 'tar'. This means that, after one and a quarter packs, or 25 cigarettes, of full-strength cigarettes, a smoker would have about 0.5 ml of 'tar' in their lungs. As already mentioned, the lungs have a capacity of 6,000ml of air, so 12,000 packs would be needed to completely fill them with 'tar'. Smoking one pack per day would accomplish that in about 33 years. This means that anyone who started smoking at age fifteen would have nothing but a thick slurry of tar oozing out of their nose and mouth by age 48. There would be no air left in his or her lungs at all, just 'tar'.

This, however, is not the end of the story. Obviously, if the lungs were completely filled with tar, then suffocation and death would be imminent. The lungs do not have to be completely filled to result in suffocation; about a cup (500 ml) is sufficient, and that is about 1,000 packs of full strength cigarettes. This could be smoked in just under three years at a pack a day. If the popular myths about cigarette 'tar' were true then every pack-a-day smoker

---

[14] http://hypertextbook.com/facts/2001/LaurenCalabrese.shtml

would be dead, from suffocation, before the end of three years.[15] This is not the case; everyone either knows or has seen an elderly smoker, or knows people who have been smoking for over three years. Even before a smoker reaches the stage of 500 ml of tar being in their lungs to kill them, they would certainly have very minimal lung capacity and would be constantly out of breath – to the point where any exercise, including walking, would be dangerous as their lungs could not provide the body with the oxygen it needs. Imagine a sponge: when dipped in water it absorbs the liquid. Imagine that same sponge dipped in tar and then in water, the tar coating would stop any water being absorbed. The same is true of the lungs with oxygen: tar would prevent oxygen passing through into the bloodstream, so death would occur instantly. All smokers would suffocate to death.

Some people attempt to counter this by saying that the body rids itself of toxins and waste. Anyone with any knowledge of tar would realise that the body cannot simply eject it – tar in the body stays there. The body can, and does, eject particles through phlegm and cilia, such as the aforementioned black produce apparent after blowing one's nose after a day in a heavily polluted area. However, actual solid tar, which is what we are led to believe accumulates in smokers lungs, is not simply ejected. If it really were so easy to get rid of, it would not have killed so many martyrs whom had it smeared on their skin to cause death by suffocation.

So, we are left with the question of 'what is the tar in cigarettes?' According to the U.S. Federal Trade Commission, tar is "total particulate matter…less nicotine and water". In other words, cigarette tar is the solid remains once the water and nicotine products have gone (through smoking, or, at least, the tobacco product being lit). It is also said the tar is "the complex of particulate matter in the smoke that is left behind on a filter after subtracting all the nicotine and moisture."[16] Interestingly, neither of these definitions supports the anti-smoking mantra that the 'tar' is the same as road tar and that it collects in the lungs.

It is important to remember that in the 1950s and 1960s the word 'tar', when used in relation to cigarettes, was used with quotations marks around it, as in this book. This was to signify that

---

[15] http://isaac.idkcomp.com/EDTORIAL/TAR.HTM?tnow=1205870771487

[16] Ashton H, Stepney R (1982) *Smoking. Psychology and Pharmacology*

it was just a term used, and that it was not actual tar like we see on the roads. Nowadays the quotation marks have been dropped and we are told it *is* the same substance; when I was in school our teacher told us they add road tar to cigarettes to make them burn easier, a statement that is clearly false.

The notion that smoking blackens the lungs can be traced back to 1948 to Ernst Wynder M.D, who will be looked at more extensively in chapter five. Wynder, then a first-year medical student in St Louis, was witness to an autopsy of a man who had died of lung cancer and he noted the lungs were blackened. The sight roused his curiosity and he looked into the background of the patient, discovering that there was no obvious exposure to air pollution but that the deceased had smoked two packs of cigarettes a day for thirty years. He linked the two and then spent his career trying to prove smoking causes cancer. However, as we are now aware, through advancements in science and our understanding of cancer, it was actually the disease itself that blackened the lungs and not the smoking. It is clear, then, that the premise smoking blackens lungs – and, indeed, causes cancer – was flawed and inaccurate from the start.

Thus, it is obvious that smoking cannot and does not leave tar in the lungs, nor does it turn the lungs black. Black lungs are the result of one or both of two things: spending years in an area with high pollution, such as a city or working as a coal miner; or cancer. In pictures comparing a non-smoker's lung with a smoker's lung, they are a non-cancerous lung and a cancerous lung, and no comparisons or assertions on lifestyle can be drawn.

# Chapter 2: Chemicals in Tobacco

There are a number of people who believe that the chemicals within tobacco products are what make smoking so harmful. Despite a lot of attention being given to these chemicals, and many attributing these chemicals as the cause of smoke-induced lung cancer, nobody knows which of the chemicals actually cause cancer. Scientists have spent hundreds of millions of dollars looking for them. Individually, some are carcinogenic and some are anti-carcinogenic, yet none account for the effects of active smoking. The total number of compounds is estimated to be 100,000, although some are unstable and exist for microseconds, and according to page 128 of the 1986 Surgeon General's Report only a few hundred have been measured at all. Indeed, the highest number of smoke particles that have been identified is from a Californian Environmental Protection Agency (EPA) report where they found 405.

The claim that there are 4,000 chemicals in cigarette smoke is almost an urban legend, misquoted from a tobacco industry scientist in the 1970s who was researching tobacco flavouring. He said there were 4,000 compounds that are produced and they were finding out which made the smoke nicer.[17] This is not the same as there being 4,000 compounds in smoke. Furthermore, many of the supposedly deadly chemicals found within tobacco smoke, such as acetone and acetaldehyde, are also exhaled by non-smokers because they are the by-product of regular metabolism.[18]

What people forget is that smoke from charcoal or candles contains many of the same components as tobacco smoke, such as carbon monoxide and formaldehyde, as well as carcinogens. In fact, a ten pound bag of charcoal produces as much smoke, and chemicals, as 160 packs of cigarettes, and an average bonfire produces as much smoke and respective chemicals as every smoker in Britain lighting up at once. As of yet, however, I have yet to hear a single cry for the banning of barbeques or indoor fires, or, indeed, people refusing to have their own coal fire or barbeque for fear of

---

[17] Roberts, D.L.(1988) "Natural Tobacco Flavor" *Recent Advances in Tobacco Science* 14: 49-81, 1988

[18] *Science.* (1992) 258: 261-265, 9th *Report On Carcinogens.* DHHS; Lawrence Taylor. *Chemical Evidence: The Forensic Expert*

contracting cancer. Similarly, a tried and tested argument from smokers is that cars emit many larger quantities of smoke and chemicals, all day every day, than cigarettes ever could. This tends to be shrugged off by non-smokers, yet it is a sound and valid argument. It is a known fact that cars in North America alone produce 3.7 billion tonnes of toxic substances – each and every year. But, like barbeques and coal fires, I have yet to hear of people avoiding driving or walking near cars because of the health risks, nor have I heard any plans to ban driving. What I am aware of, though, is that there is now major concern about the state of our planet, in part due to the fumes of fires and vehicle pollution; it is amusing that people believe exhaust fumes have the power to destroy their planet but will do no harm to their lungs or the rest of their body.

One of the fastest ways a person can kill themselves is carbon monoxide poisoning, by running a hosepipe from the car exhaust into a window, leading to death within minutes. A lot of people now have carbon monoxide detectors in their homes so they know if there is a CO leak, as it can cause poisoning or death. So, then, everyone is more than aware of the dangers of CO and where it can be found, yet people are more than happy to continue their lives without worry. Are we really to believe that a small amount of tobacco is to kill us with chemicals, when we are surrounded by the same chemicals each and every day of our lives? Perhaps the American comedian and social critic Bill Hicks summed it up perfectly: "I smoke. If this bothers anyone, I suggest looking at the world in which we live and shutting your mouth."

Consider for a moment where else we find chemicals, and toxic chemicals at that. Tap water is chlorinated and often fluoridated, both of which have been shown to be extremely dangerous and damaging to the body. There is more benzene in a glass of tap water in certain geographical areas than in a cigarette, and there are now massive levels of chemicals in water due to pollution and pharmaceutical drugs being flushed down the toilet. A video on Youtube explains the EPA's troubles with America's water and the extent of its contamination,[19] and certain areas in

---

[19] http://www.youtube.com/watch?v=TVZRD5gZoHE

America have Benzene in the water.[20] Crops are sprayed with pesticides which, as any nutritionist will explain, lowers the body's immune system and have the capacity to harm you – pesticides are, after all, designed to kill living organisms. Many household cleaners carry large warnings telling us to avoid contact with the skin or eyes, and to seek medical attention if said product is ingested. At the same time, though, we are permitted to spray these products onto our surfaces and then make contact with the surface, or eat food from the area.

We consume large quantities of chemicals everyday of our lives, with things we consider 'necessities' such as shampoo, conditioner, hand cream, body lotion, moisturiser, sun cream lotion, and make-up. We are now starting to see a consequence from all these chemicals: make-up has been linked to cancers, especially breast cancer in women, and the water supply in the United Kingdom is contaminated with large quantities of the female hormone oestrogen as well as chemotherapy drugs and Diazepam, a psychiatric drug.[21] The U.K. watchdog has found benzene in soft drinks[22] and similar findings emerged in numerous American states, as much as 27 times the safe limit:[23]

> Test results for other drinks also revealed the presence of highly elevated benzene levels. One cola drink the FDA tested was contaminated at 138 ppb, 27 times the 5 ppb tap water limit, and a fruit drink had 95 ppb. Orange and grapefruit juice also had benzene at levels well above FDA's 5 ppb level of concern.

---

[20] http://www.watersystemscouncil.org/vaiwebdocs/wscdocs/1463522benzene.pdf

[21] Report commissioned by Drinking Water Inspectorate (DWI), published in *The Telegraph* Jan 13 2008

[22] http://www.beveragedaily.com/news/ng.asp?n=66160-benzene-soft-drinks-fsa March 1st 2006 *Britain's food safety watchdog says initial tests on 230 soft drinks show benzene levels above the UK limit for water*

[23] http://www.flex-news-food.com/pages/2363/Benzene/Beverages/FDA/Food-Safety/Frozen/Fruit/Tea/environmental-working-group-fda-data-undercut-public-safety-assurances-top-agency-official.html

Further to all of this is the fact that our oceans are being overloaded with plastic as a result of our dependence on the product.[24] [25] NaturalNews reported that:

The plastic pieces, whether mistaken for food or so microscopic as to be unavoidable, are consumed by seabirds and fish, which in turn make it to our dinner plates. This can have disastrous consequences for food webs and human health. Many of these chemicals have hormone disrupting properties that affect both animals and humans.

Plastic itself has been linked to a variety of very serious health problems, for example it was noted that over 80% of the male small mouth bass in the Potomac were growing eggs.[26] In addition, a study conducted by Dr. Shanna Swan, published in *Environmental Health Perspectives* in August 2005, found that "pregnant women with higher urine concentrations of some phthalates were more likely to give birth to sons with 'phthalate syndrome'—incomplete male genital development—a disorder previously seen only in lab rats."[27] The lead researcher said:

These changes in male infants, associated with prenatal exposure to some of the same phthalate metabolites that cause similar alterations in male rodents, suggest that commonly used phthalates may undervirilize humans as well as rodents.[28]

Yet we continue to use plastic daily for a variety of purposes and little or nothing is mentioned from the authorities about the possible health effects. There are also plenty more products on the

---

[24] http://www.naturalnews.com/022885.html *A swirling, floating garbage dump in the North Pacific Ocean twice the size of the United States has been noticed in recent years and is growing at a swift pace*

[25] *Best Life Magazine*, February 20th 2007

[26] *Common Ground* March 2007 http://commongroundmag.com/2007/03/plastichassle.html

[27] Ibid.

[28] http://www.ehponline.org/members/2005/8100/8100.html

market which we perhaps should be worried about. For example, our waters are so contaminated that fish have very high levels of mercury[29] which is known to cause nerve and kidney damage, and Teflon has a large, and growing, body of evidence against it highlighting links between its use and cancer, as well as the discovery that there are actually chemicals present on earth since the production of Teflon that did not exist beforehand.[30] Additionally, aluminium has long been linked to Alzheimer's disease, in fact there was mention years ago about not using cookware made of it, however such apparatus continues to be made of aluminium and it can also be found in a range of other products including deodorants and antiperspirants – none of which carry a health warning of any description.

Should we be asking why not? More than likely, we are all aware of the answer to the question, so perhaps what we should really be doing is asking the question loudly enough with the hope that things may change – or at least be explained.

According to MCS-Global:

> Toxic effects of chemical agents are often not well understood or appreciated by health care providers and the general public. Some chemicals, such as asbestos, vinyl chloride and lead, are known to cause human disease. Other studies suggest that increases in the incidence of some cancers, asthma, and developmental disorders also can be attributed to chemical exposure, particularly in young children. More than 80,000 chemicals have been developed, used, distributed, and discarded into the environment over the past 50 years. The majority of them have not been tested for potential toxic effects in humans or wildlife. Some of these chemicals are commonly in air, water, food, homes, work places, and communities. Whereas the toxicity of one chemical may be incompletely understood, an understanding of the impacts from exposure to mixtures of

---

[29] Ken Cook, President of the Environmental Working Group. Article online at http://articles.mercola.com/sites/articles/archive/2001/04/25/mercury-fish-part-one.aspx

[30] http://www.eartheasy.com/article_teflon_toxicity.htm

chemicals is even more deficient. Chemicals may have opposing, additive, or even synergistic effects.

MCS-Global use Roundup as an example, it defines the product thusly:

> Roundup is a common herbicide used extensively by local governments to control weeds in our streets and parks. Many people use Roundup in their home gardens. The active ingredient in Roundup is called glyphosate but there are numerous different brands of herbicide containing glyphosate that are marketed under different names

and go on to say:

> Monsanto, the original manufacturers of Roundup, claim that their product "poses no danger to human health when used according to label directions" and that "no special protective clothing or equipment is required when spraying Roundup". But can these safety claims be trusted?

Directly following this they list conditions that Roundup has been linked to, including cancer, reproductive problems, birth defects, asthma in children, skin diseases, multiple chemical sensitivity, and neurobehavioural disorders.[31] Clearly, then, chemicals *can* and *do* affect us greatly. The most important thing, though, is perspective – whilst these things are bad for us and can cause serious problems, a little exposure will be fine. It is for this reason that the people most at risk are those working with such products, as opposed to those using them now and again in real world conditions.

Phillip Morris International, probably the largest tobacco company in the world and manufacturer of the most popular brand of cigarettes, Marlboro, have information on the ingredients and amounts of each ingredient in their cigarettes.[32] Whilst there is, indeed, an extensive list of additives, the first thing to point out is that not all of them are artificial chemicals. For example, water is

---

[31] http://www.mcs-global.org/Chemicals.htm

[32] http://www.pmintl-technical-product-information.com/aspx/country.aspx?CountryName=GR

12

also added as is, in certain brands, sugar and certain oils such as coriander. Secondly, whilst there are chemical additives, they make up a minute amount of the cigarette: most artificial chemicals and additives constitute 0.0001% of the cigarette. Given the size and weight of a cigarette, it is very obvious that 0.0001% amounts to practically nothing. To give a more accurate example, in the brand Marlboro Red there are 0.035 milligrams of flavourings – both natural and artificial – per cigarette. Smoking twenty cigarettes a day still only produces 0.7 mg, not even one thousandth of a gram. To put this into context, the Queen's nose on a British coin weighs a gram, yet it is over a thousand times more than the natural and artificial flavourings present in a cigarette. Furthermore, there is not a single ingredient in tobacco products that is not approved for use, nor is there a single chemical or additive that we do not get from other sources including food and water. Ammonia, for example, is present in fertilisers. It is also important to remember that what is in a cigarette is not necessarily what is in the smoke – when something is oxidised the chemical structure changes and an unpleasant substance could become quite harmless.

One of the most popular counter-arguments to this is the idea that the chemicals become more harmful when burnt, a notion that seems sound in theory but in practice has not been demonstrated. As a matter of fact, animals are routinely used in testing chemicals to see how they affect them and could possibly affect humans. Rodents, in particular, are very similar in physiology to us and what is bad for them tends to be bad for us, and vice versa. However, to this day, no one has managed to induce lung cancer in animals with tobacco products,[33] despite using tobacco products sold for commercial use i.e. with all the additives and chemicals present. We will look at the studies in greater detail in chapter five. What they have done, however, is to use tobacco extracts and cause skin cancer by placing the extract on the animals skin. Whilst this is used to scare people, in actuality any product that irritates the skin can cause skin cancer, and it is not tobacco but selected extracts which are used.

---

[33] "Minnesota vs. Tobacco" court case, 1998, experts stated that "although there had been many experiments with animals, trying to induce lung cancer by forcing the animals to inhale tobacco smoke, all the experiments had failed."

What has been shown, though, is that other chemicals are incredibly deadly but are marketed as safe. The artificial sweetener aspartame is a very good example. Aspartame, a.k.a NutraSweet, was not approved until 1981. The Food and Drink Administration (FDA) refused to approve it because it had caused seizures and brain tumours in laboratory animals, and they continued to refuse its approval until Ronald Reagan became President of the USA. and fired the FDA commissioner. The Bressler Report compared all available raw data and summary data against the manufacturer's FDA submission and found missing raw data, as well as errors and discrepancies in what available data there was. The FDA investigated Searle and published a scathing 76 page report uncovering the discrepancies, inconsistencies, and evidence of fabrication of records in Searle's lab work. They also performed their own autopsies on the remaining corpses of the experimental rats and found a large number of pathological conditions which were caused by the aspartame but not reported by Searle in their analysis of the results. The Bressler report was obtained by a health activist, Barbara Mullarkey, using the Freedom of Information Act. The FDA has since passed into the control of persons with economic and political ties to the new owners of the GD Searle Company – the notorious Monsanto Corporation, makers of poisons and political intriguers who are number one on the list of companies being watched by environmentalists worldwide for their campaign of destruction of the environment and disregard for human health in the name of corporate greed. The FDA, prior to turning the report over to Mullarkey, blanked out some of the attached charts and memos, as if they were some sort of state secrets. [34]

In 1981 Reagan appointed Dr. Arthur Hull Hayes as the FDA commissioner, who then approved aspartame for use in dry goods.[35] In 1983 the FDA approved aspartame to be used in carbonated beverages and in 1993 approved it for use in other beverages, baked goods and confections. Finally, in 1996 the FDA removed all restrictions thus allowing aspartame to be used in all foods. We can see the deceit and inner-workings that allowed

---

[34] http://www.presidiotex.com/bressler/index.html

[35] http://archive.gao.gov/d28t5/133460.pdf

aspartame to be approved and marketed without a warning. However, it gets worse.

Methanol/wood alcohol is a well known deadly poison. It was, in fact, the poison that caused some 'skid row' alcoholics to lose their sight, and in some cases killed them. Methanol is gradually released in the small intestine when the methyl group of aspartame encounter the enzyme Chymotrypsin. The absorption of methanol into the body is sped up considerably when free methanol is ingested, and free methanol is created from aspartame when it is heated to over 86°F, or 30°C. Such an occurrence would take place often given that aspartame is now contained in baked goods and other foods that will be heated. Methanol then breaks down into formic acid and formaldehyde[36] in the body – formaldehyde being a well known, deadly neurotoxin. An EPA assessment states that methanol

> is considered a cumulative poison due to the low rate of excretion once it is absorbed. In the body, methanol is oxidised to formaldehyde and formic acid; both of these metabolites are toxic.

The recommended limit of consumption is less than 7.8 mg per day, however a one litre beverage containing aspartame, such as Diet Coke, contains about 56 mg of methanol. People ingesting a lot of products with aspartame can find themselves consuming up to 250 mg of methanol a day – 32 times the EPA limit. The soldiers of Desert Storm were provided with large amounts of beverages sweetened with aspartame which had been heated to over 86°F in the Saudi Arabian sun, and many of the soldiers returned home with numerous disorders similar to what has been witnessed in those who have been poisoned by formaldehyde. It is very possible that the methanol in the drinks the soldiers consumed was a contributing factor in these illnesses.

Whilst it is true that fruit juices and alcoholic beverages contain small amounts of methanol, it is important to remember than the methanol in natural products never appears alone, rather, in every case, ethanol is present. Ethanol is an antidote for methanol toxicity in humans, as such cancelling out the damage that

---

[36] Trocho, C. *et. al* (1998). "*Formaldehyde derived from dietary aspartame binds to tissue components in vivo*".

the methanol could cause. However, because aspartame is synthetic it does not contain any ethanol.

In February 1994, the U.S. Department of Health and Human Services released the listing of adverse reactions reported to the FDA. Aspartame accounted for more than 75% of all adverse reactions reported to the FDA's Adverse Reaction Monitoring System (ARMS). This is a conservative figure, though, as the FDA admits that less than 1% of those who have problems with something they consume ever report it to the FDA. What this means, then, is that the 10,000 complaints they received could represent nearer to a million.

Of course, since aspartame has been approved there have been numerous studies emerging to show it is safe. Needless to say, though, a harmful product does not become safe merely because interests have become vested. All that changes is the interests of people, and this skews results. In other words, those with financial interest in aspartame have generated studies assuring people of its safety.

Some may point out I have contradicted myself by highlighting that all the additives in cigarette smoke are approved for consumption, and then following that with evidence of a legal and widely consumed product that can be damaging to the human body. My point is that, in laboratory testing, tobacco products have never reliably caused cancer or death to an animal, yet there are products on the market that have. Furthermore, the added chemicals present within cigarettes make up such a small amount of the cigarette they barely exist within it. Even smoking fifty cigarettes a day would not give much exposure to the chemicals, certainly not enough to cause any damage to the body.

Let us take a look at some of the chemicals within tobacco that receive the most negative attention:

Anti-smokers are fond of informing others that carbon monoxide kills people and depletes oxygen within the body. Like oxygen, carbon monoxide combines chemically with the haemoglobin in red blood cells, but, unlike oxygen, the CO is not released, instead it stays there until the cell expires and is replaced by a new one. Each molecule of CO takes up a 'slot' where oxygen might otherwise be carried to where it is needed, but one molecule of CO does not destroy the oxygen carrying capacity of the entire cell as haemoglobin is a large molecule whose purpose is to carry many oxygen molecules. It is true, though, that very large amounts of CO will displace enough oxygen that suffocation can result. What must be remembered is there is no danger that this will occur through smoking, because there is not nearly enough carbon monoxide present. As stated before in this chapter, there is far more CO from vehicles than any tobacco product. Actually, the biggest CO danger comes from home appliances and the federal Centers for Disease Control and Prevention says:

> Carbon monoxide is the leading cause of poisoning deaths in the United States. As many as 5,000 people die of it each year, and another 10,000 are stricken ill enough to miss at least one day of work. The gas takes its victims silently and insidiously, seeping into their lungs from furnaces, chimneys, heaters, large appliances, automobiles on a nearby roadway or even a neighbouring apartment [37]

Thus, whilst carbon monoxide can be destructive, the quantities present within tobacco smoke are too minute to harm the human body. Researchers have recently discovered that small amounts of carbon monoxide appear to have a beneficial effect on the body which may help prevent brain damage following a stroke.[38] The Bio-Medicine website states:

> The Hopkins team found that low amounts of inhaled carbon monoxide reduced brain damage by as much as 62.2 percent in mice with strokes induced by briefly blocking an artery to one side of the brain. The researchers believe that CO can protect nerve cells from damage.

And the study author, Sylvain Dor, had this to say:

> CO is made naturally by the body and can serve a protective function under various circumstances. The idea for our experiment was to see if external CO could have a similar effect.

The study concluded:

---

[37] Planet Rx

[38] http://www.bio-medicine.org/medicine-news-1/Small-Doses-of-Carbon-Monoxide-Might-Help-Stroke-Victims-32386-1/

The protective effect was evident in mice treated at both one and three hours after stroke. This is an important point, because "many stroke victims will not receive immediate treatment" Dor said.

Given these findings, an interesting study would be to compare smokers and non-smokers following a stroke, to determine if there is any difference in brain damage or recovery rates. Nonetheless, it is very apparent that low-levels of carbon monoxide, like the level in tobacco smoke, do not pose a health threat.

Formaldehyde is a very well known chemical and has been mentioned in this chapter already. The EPA has Formaldehyde down as a potential carcinogen, meaning it is not yet known, or is not conclusively proven, that it causes cancer. It is, however, a known neurotoxin. It is without wonder that people worry about it being in tobacco smoke. However, before getting too concerned, we must look at the big picture. A cigarette, on average, delivers 20-90 micrograms in mainstream smoke and up to 700 micrograms in side stream smoke. However, space heaters and gas ranges release 20,000–40,000 micrograms *per hour*. Formaldehyde is also used extensively in wood finish, glue, fabric coating, insulation, and many other places. In mobile homes, concentrations have been measured in excess of 5,000 micrograms per cubic metre. In 'non-sick' buildings, the typical level is 50 mg per cubic metre, the same concentration as side stream smoke – 40-50 micrograms per metre cubed. Comparatively, the official safe level is 1,500 micrograms per metre cubed.[39] It is worth noting in passing that formaldehyde is not added to cigarettes, but is produced naturally from the combustion when the tobacco is lit.

Benzene and toluene are perhaps next to formaldehyde in the sense of being seen as the scourge of tobacco additives, and they are mentioned as potential environmental tobacco smoke (ETS) carcinogens. They are associated with leukaemia, but leukaemia has never been linked to active smoking let alone second-hand smoke. Benzene, toluene and other aromatics found in the air are primarily found in gasoline, or petrol, but also in copy machines, glue, paint and other such sources. Typically, concentrations in indoor air are 2-20 micrograms per metre cubed, the same as in environmental tobacco smoke. When filling a car with fuel, a person

---

[39] Ibid

is exposed to concentrations 50-100 times higher. The official safety level for benzene is 30,000 micrograms per metre cubed, and for toluene 375,000 micrograms per metre cubed – over a thousand times that found in ETS in most situations.[40] Like formaldehyde, benzene is produced whenever carbon-rich materials undergo incomplete combustion, so is therefore not an additive in cigarettes but a naturally-occurring substance.

Benzo[a]pyrene is an interesting chemical. In 1996 researchers claimed they had found the exact way in which smoking caused lung cancer: by the Benzo[a]pyrene (BAP) in cigarette smoke damaging the p53 gene. The article in question will be looked at further in chapter five, but firstly BAP needs to be examined in a little more detail. Typically, a room with no smoke has .1-1 nanograms per metre cubed, and .3-1.5 nanograms per metre cubed with ETS. Outside air, with heavy traffic, has 1-3 nanograms per metre cubed. A nanogram is a billionth of a gram, an unfathomable amount. Interestingly, our primary exposure comes from food and water rather than air. It is estimated that we take in 1,000–5,000 nanograms per day from the air, whereas tap water contains 1-10 nanograms per litre, and one piece of charcoal-broiled meat delivers about 2,500 nanograms. BAP is produced by the combustion of vegetation and fossil fuels, and most of our intake comes from burnt food. Despite this, though, the richest source is leafy green vegetables, which pick it up from the air as a result of burnt vegetation and fossil fuels etc., which is the same way water is contaminated.

Professor Pybus, of the University of Newcastle-upon-Tyne, has shown that in England the BAP in coal smoke per year was 375 tonnes, whereas all the tobacco smoke in the country in one year was a measly 8 lbs. Additionally, Dr. Paul Kotin, an American pathologist, calculated that the BAP in 350,000 cigarettes is the equivalent to one minute's emission from a diesel truck. So, there is so much BAP in the environment already as for smoking to be entirely incidental. Finally, American researchers conducted a study whereby workers were exposed to the equivalent of 700 cigarettes a day for six years. At the end of the study an official of the American Cancer Society stated to a U.S. Congressional Committee on November 13th 1969 that: "It is most unlikely that Benzo[a]pyrene has anything to do with lung cancer." Those in

---

[40] Ibid

Britain may remember a short while ago the "Smoke is Poison"[41] campaign by Cancer Research U.K.. The campaign attempted to show tobacco smoke as poisonous because of the chemicals contained within it, and they highlighted six: benzene, arsenic, hydrogen cyanide, formaldehyde, cadmium and polonium. The campaign explained how deadly the chemicals are, but forgot two important things: the incredibly small quantity present within tobacco smoke, and that each and every one is present in foods – they are common chemicals found in fertilisers, the soil and other places. Benzene exists in exhaust fumes, and there are 25 American states whose water supply is contaminated with large quantities of arsenic. Polonium-210 is present in the soil, and is therefore in every product grown in the ground.

Finally, we will look at nicotine. Nicotine is either very misunderstood or just a victim of propaganda. Nicotine is not a carcinogen as some suggest, nor is it only in the tobacco plant. According to a study conducted by Norden, with researchers including members of the National Food Administration of Sweden and Danish Veterinary and Food Administration,

> Nicotine has been detected in potatoes, tomatoes, eggplants, and sweet peppers, all food plants and members of the large family Solanaceae. The nicotine levels were extremely low in fresh potatoes, tomatoes and sweet peppers, below 10 µg/kg. Somewhat higher levels, but still very low amounts, were found in fresh eggplant fruits (up to 100 µg/kg). Processed products contained equivalent or slightly higher levels of nicotine than fresh products (up to 34 µg/kg). [42]

One study[43] showed that eating a normal portion (4.9 oz) of mashed potatoes produced the same amount of nicotine in a workers blood as 4 hours spent in a smoky bar, and a long lunch with a smoking friend can be equalled by a third of an ounce of eggplant. Whilst not carcinogenic, nicotine is toxic in the right dose. However, caffeine, too, is poisonous and a gram of pure caffeine

---

[41] http://info.cancerresearchuk.org/healthyliving/smokeispoison/

[42] http://www.norden.org/pub/ebook/2003-531.pdf

[43] Domino et al, Med. Sci. Res, (1993) *Relevance of Nicotine Content of Common Vegetables To The Identification of Passive Tobacco Smokers*,

can kill a person. Furthermore, apples contain cyanide, strawberries contain benzene, and there are over 10,000 naturally occurring poisons in the food items that we eat everyday. Whilst nicotine itself is poisonous, the amount found in cigarettes is far from the amount required – nor is it the concentrated form required – to kill someone. If it were, a lot of smokers would be dead or in hospital due to nicotine poisoning.[44]

On the subject of chemicals, and the criticism that is directed at tobacco because of them, coffee is an interesting substance to look at. Scientists have identified 1,000 different chemicals in a single cup of coffee. Whilst this alone may be shocking, what is even more so is that only twenty-two of these 1,000 have ever been tested in animal cancer studies – meaning 978 have not. Even more noteworthy is the fact that of the twenty-two tested chemicals, seventeen were found to be carcinogenic.

Carcinogens are found in many foods – as are offsetting cancer-fighting chemicals – but in small quantities. If we wanted to avoid all carcinogens, we would have to stop eating altogether. But there are 10 mg of known carcinogens in a single cup of coffee. To put that into perspective, 10 mg is probably more than all the synthetic pesticide residues you could get from eating non-organic food for an entire year. In one cup.[45]

In the 1964 Surgeon General's report there was a committee of ten scientists who were picked from 150 scientists and physicians. All ten of the scientists were heavily weighted towards government agencies and large organisations that were active in public relations, with a low representation from the scientific community. Interestingly, there were no statisticians on the committee, despite the fact that statistical expertise is imperative to a proper analysis of the epidemiological studies which formed a large part of the so-called evidence that was studied (in 1965 K.A. Brownlee, a prominent statistician of the University of Chicago,

---

[44] Source for some of the information on specific chemicals: Huber et al Smoke *and Mirrors*, Regulation: 16:3:44 (1993) Original source: Guerin, Jenkins & Tomkins, "*The Chemistry of ETS: Composition Measurement*", Chelsea, Michigan; Lewis Publishers (1992)

[45] Primedia, Intertec (2003) http://wiki.answers.com/Q/ How_many_chemicals_are_in_one_cup_of_coffee

wrote a damning review on the Report, which we will look at later[46]).

The committee discovered that, according to their work, the most potent carcinogen present in tobacco smoke is Benzo[a]pyrene (p27 of the Report). However, despite what has been mentioned already about BAP, the committee found their own discrepancy – they said that there is four times the amount of BAP in cigar smoke as in cigarette smoke, and ten times the amount of cigarette smoke in pipe smoke. Yet, oddly, they found both cigar and pipe smoke to be essentially innocent of causing lung cancer and concluded that pipe smokers live longer than non-smokers. There is the argument that it is because of inhalation of cigarette smoke compared to non-inhalation of cigar and pipe smoke. Multiple studies have been conducted to test the validity of this notion, which are examined later in the book; it is interesting to see how even the most potent carcinogen in tobacco smoke does not present a consistent supporting argument that smoking is harmful.

Should we be worried about chemicals? The short answer is yes. The long answer is yes, but not all of them. While the chemicals contained within cigarettes are not good for us, the simple fact remains that the quantities within which they exist are so small they will not be causing any damage to us.

---

[46] Brownlee. K.A. (1965) *A Review of "Smoking and Health"* J. Amer. Statist. Ass. 60

# Chapter 3: Smoking and Socio-Economic Status (SES)

The issue of social class is one that is exceptionally important but criminally overlooked by today's health community, and indeed the public at large. There is a very definite class-divide when it comes to tobacco users, with most cigarette smokers tending to come from the lower classes, and pipe and cigar smokers tending to be from the upper classes. It is no secret, of course, that those from the lower classes have less money, more physical and often more dangerous jobs (such as factory work or working with chemicals), worse lifestyles and diets than those in the upper classes, and tend to have poorer healthcare. On the other hand, those in the upper classes lead more relaxed lives, eat better food and have healthier lifestyles. Statistically, then, showing that cigarette smokers contract lung cancer more than non-smokers really shows that people from lower social classes are more likely to get lung cancer. (Even farther back in history when cigarette smoking was more equal amongst all classes, the other lifestyle factors would have existed, probably to a higher degree as hygiene and living conditions have improved drastically over the years.) Actually, people with a lower socio-economic status are more likely to die younger anyway, lung cancer or not. This is something the anti-smokers overlook, deliberately or not I do not know, but the fact is the issue of class and illness is often neglected, which is jumping the gun somewhat.

In their book *The Health Trap* Richard Dorsett and Alan Marsh look at smoking and poverty, and we are told in the blurb that:

> Smoking has become more and more concentrated among Britain's poorest families...The poorest group – Britain's 1.7 million lone parent families – smoke most...Among the large group of lone parents who rely on council housing and social security benefits, more than three-quarters smoke...Lone parents who smoke pay nearly £300 million a year back to the Treasury.

Marsh and Dorsett say in the book:

> No trough of poverty was lower and no peak of smoking was higher than at the social location occupied by growing numbers of lone parents. It may as well be said now that if

23

you are a poorly educated lone parent living in council accommodation and receiving Income Support, as so many lone parents are, then your chances of being a smoker are over 80 per cent. This in a world where now only 25 per cent of young women smoke and among the better off young women, fewer than a fifth smoke.[47]

Firstly, let us look at a table[48] of the mean income of smokers and non-smokers in British pounds per week. The table gives data which shows that the average income of a smoker is lower than that of a non-smoker:

| Smoker/non-smoker | 1991 | 1993 | 1994 |
|---|---|---|---|
| Smokers | 95 | 105 | 105 |
| Non-smokers | 113 | 128 | 127 |

The figures speak for themselves and show a significant difference in pay – not a huge difference, but significant nonetheless. What is particularly interesting about the figures is that smokers earn less than non-smokers in all three years of study, and in fact the difference increases as the years go on, showing it is not an anomaly for one year only. On page forty of the book is another table, this one showing the indicators of welfare by smoker:

| | 1991 | | 1993 | | 1994 | |
|---|---|---|---|---|---|---|
| | S | NS | S | NS | S | NS |
| No. food items unable to afford | 1.1 | 0.6 | 1.0 | 0.7 | 0.9 | 0.8 |
| No. clothing items unable to afford | 2.7 | 1.7 | 2.9 | 1.8 | 2.7 | 2.1 |

---

[47] Dorsett, R; Marsh, A. (1998) *The Health Trap. Poverty, Smoking and Lone Parenthood* Athenaeum Press (p 20)

[48] Ibid.

| No. durable goods unable to afford | 3.1 | 2.4 | 3.4 | 2.2 | 2.6 | 2.2 |
|---|---|---|---|---|---|---|
| No. problem debts | 0.9 | 0.6 | 0.8 | 0.6 | 0.9 | 0.7 |
| Any children's needs can't afford to meet? (%) | 52 | 39 | 56 | 34 | 51 | 35 |
| Any own needs can't afford to meet? (%) | 54 | 41 | 62 | 45 | 65 | 44 |
| Index of relative material hardship | 1.9 | 1.1 | 2.0 | 1.2 | 1.7 | 1.5 |
| *Weighted n* | 493 | 446 | 410 | 429 | 430 | 424 |

The information following the table informs us that the researchers, Marsh and Mckay (1994), define those scoring three or above as suffering severe hardship. Of the two times there is a score of over three both occur in the smokers category and, similarly, the ones near three but below it are in the smokers category. The non-smokers scores tend to be much lower, indicating less financial troubles.

Following this table is a distribution of the index, in another table, to show whether smokers or non-smokers are more likely to be in severe hardship. The table is included here:

| Relative Material Hardship Score | 1991 | | 1993 | | 1994 | |
|---|---|---|---|---|---|---|
| | S | NS | S | NS | S | NS |
| 0 | 24 | 47 | 25 | 40 | 31 | 44 |
| 1 | 23 | 20 | 17 | 27 | 21 | 19 |

| 2 | 20 | 15 | 21 | 16 | 17 | 18 |
|---|----|----|----|----|----|----|
| 3 | 17 | 11 | 17 | 11 | 13 | 10 |
| 4 | 10 | 6 | 12 | 5 | 12 | 7 |
| 5 | 5 | 1 | 6 | 1 | 5 | 3 |
| 6 | 2 | 0 | 2 | 0 | 1 | 0 |
| 3 or more | 34 | 18 | 37 | 17 | 31 | 20 |
| *Weighted n* | 493 | 446 | 410 | 429 | 430 | 424 |

The information given below the table says:

> As expected, smokers appear worse off than non-smokers. A much higher proportion of non-smokers have a score of zero on the relative material hardship index, while smokers are more prevalent among those households with a score of three or more. The pattern for scores of one and two is more mixed. Approximately a third of all smoking lone parents are in severe hardship, nearly twice the figure for non-smokers.

So, there is no denying that smokers are most prevalent in the lower classes, and it is no secret; nor is there a shortage of evidence to show that those in the lower classes have worse health than those in higher classes. For instance, a 1991 Canadian study showed that people with a high social status had a 1.9% chance of suffering a major psychological depression; people in a medium social class had a 4.5% chance, and people in the lowest social classes had a 12.4% chance.[49] Furthermore, a 1990 study found relationships between smoking and levels of education in America,[50] as shown in the following table:

---

[49] Murphy, et al (1991) *Depression and Anxiety in Relation to Social Status* Archives of General Psychiatry

[50] Winkelby et al., (1990) *Social Class Disparities in Risk Factors for Disease: Eight year prevalence patterns by level of education* Preventive Medicine: 19:1.

| Years of Education | Males | Females |
|---|---|---|
| Less than 13 | 41 | 36 |
| 13 – 15 | 30 | 24 |
| 16 | 25 | 15 |
| 16 or more | 18 | 17 |

We can compare this with a 1973 study which correlates morbidity with educational levels:[51]

Ratio of Observed to Expected Deaths, U.S., ages 21-65:

| Years of Education | Males | Females |
|---|---|---|
| 16 + | 0.70 | 0.78 |
| 13 – 15 | 0.85 | 0.82 |
| 12 | 0.91 | 0.87 |
| 9 – 11 | 1.03 | 0.91 |
| 8 | 1.07 | 1.08 |
| 5 – 7 | 1.13 | 1.18 |
| Less than 5 | 1.17 | 1.60 |

What these figures show is that people in lower classes tend to smoke more, and also tend to die younger. While anti-smokers jump to the conclusion that this is because of smoking, that is entirely premature given the multifaceted elements differentially impacting those in lower social classes. To assume that these have no bearing on health would be ridiculous as it would ultimately mean smoking is the only factor that negatively impacts health. Furthermore, as mentioned in chapter two, pipe smokers tend to live longer than even non-smokers, something most people will find incredibly puzzling. Of course, many will point out that pipe and cigar smokers do not generally inhale, whilst cigarette smokers do. However, there are three problems with this theory: firstly, there is

---

[51] Kitigawa & Hauser (1973) *Differential mortality in the United States: A study in socioeconomic epidemiology* Harvard University Press.

more tobacco and more smoke in pipes and cigars and thus more exposure. As such, life expectancy could decrease from oral cancers, not to mention that, if cigarette smoke can apparently affect the pancreas and bladder (as we are told) then the effects pipe and cigar smoke would also not only be confined to the mouth; secondly, and arguably most importantly, Doll and Hill conducted a study on inhalation and non-inhalation and found there to be an inverse effect: those who inhaled suffered lower rates of lung cancer than non-inhalers. This study is explained in chapter five, but that point is relevant here. Thirdly and finally, pipes and cigars produce a very large amount of concentrated second-hand smoke, which the smoker ends up inhaling as he or she breathes. If, as we are told, second-hand smoke can be responsible for thousands of deaths then it stands to reason that pipe and cigar smokers would suffer a lot of smoking-related diseases.

The smoking and social class issue has also been recognised by Heather Ashton and Rob Stepney in their book *Smoking, Psychology and Pharmacology*[52] as, on page eleven, they state:

> However, whilst the sex difference has become less pronounced, a difference according to social class has emerged...In certain working-class areas smoking is apparently still nearly ubiquitous. A report in the Observer Magazine described life on the Creggan Estate in Londonderry, where stress factors may also be presumed to play a part in the prevalence of smoking.

They then include the excerpt from the *Observer Magazine*, which is included here also:

> In the poorer houses just about everybody smokes, ashtrays are full of butts. It is a place where it is still an act of hospitality to offer a pack or actually toss cigarettes round the room on the assumption that everyone smokes. Finger tips are yellow-brown with nicotine, and clouds of smoke eddy round the television screen.[53]

---

[52] Ashton, H; Stepney, R (1982) *Smoking, Psychology and Pharmacology* Tavistock Publications

[53] *Observer Magazine*, 31 December 1978

What we can deduce, then, is that there is simply no escaping the fact that cigarette smokers are most prevalent in the lower classes, and there is no shortage of evidence to show, conclusively, that poorer people are more likely to suffer from a variety of health problems, as the above study on depression shows. Whilst these references are quite old, this is to show that the classes have been studied for a long time, primarily because of the health situation and, as a trip to the library will show, the smoking rates.

A more recent study, from 2000 by Trinder et al,[54] published in the *British Medical Journal,* also looked at smoking and social class, with the hypothesis that smoking causes respiratory illness. The study has its flaws, for instance the survey sample was relatively small at 4,237 participants, and its methodology was a questionnaire. However, the results found that:

> Social class is linked to the severity of respiratory symptoms, independently of smoking. Although the need to reduce and quit smoking in manual class households remains a crucial preventive issue, other mechanisms by which social class differences may influence symptom occurrence and severity need to be explored.

This conclusion shows that not only is the link between smoking and respiratory illness grossly overstated, but also that there has been very little research looking at what other causes there may be despite the main factor seeming to be social class.

Despite time passing, the lower social classes still make up the main body of cigarette smokers. Tobacco companies have been banned from advertising for many years, so what is causing people to start smoking? A 2006 report[55] found that parents who smoke often pass their habit on to their children of the same sex – meaning fathers may pass their habit on to their sons, and mothers to daughters. The report also looked at single parents and found that the results still applied, except that offspring of either sex were influenced by their single parent. Statistically, single parents tend to

---

[54] http://jech.bmj.com/cgi/content/abstract/54/5/340

[55] http://ftp.iza.org/dp2279.pdf

be from the lower classes. Thus, recent data still supports existing data that cigarette smokers are mostly from the lower social classes.

In keeping with the above paragraph's point, a 2006 article on a health news website[56] reported a study looking at social status, smoking and death rates among men, saying:

> A recent study has shed some light on smoking, social status and death rates among men. The findings suggest that death rates among male smokers of a lower social/economic status are twice as high as men of a higher social/economic status.

The study appeared in the *Guardian*, a neutral and respected British newspaper, and the aforementioned health website links to the article. In that same year the *Guardian* published another article on social class, reporting a study which found the lower your socio-economic status the faster you age.[57] The researchers even stated that they ruled out smoking as a possible reason for the outcome. Again, then, recent data supports older data about the impact on health of belonging at the bottom of the social chain.

This realisation of the importance of social status no doubt also accounts for the idea that smoking causes wrinkled and aging skin and other 'ailments'. Such things are not from smoking, but from poor lifestyle which people easily attribute to smoking because it is a very common factor amongst those people, or at least it is the one visible factor that people can see and then blame. What causes these people to be at more risk is not known entirely, given the number of possible factors such as stress, lifestyle, dangerous jobs, poor diet etc., but what we *can* say, based on this evidence, is that showing cigarette smokers to have a statistically increased risk of lung cancer shows nothing when we consider who the bulk of the cigarette smokers are. In short, those figures really tell us that people with a low socio-economic status are at higher risk than people with a high social-economic status – smokers or not.

---

[56] http://www.healthyforms.com/health-news/2006/07/smoking-and-social-status.php

[57] http://www.guardian.co.uk/science/2006/jul/20/lifeandhealth.medicineandhealth

# Chapter 4: Detection Bias

The idea of detection bias is one that many people are oblivious to, as there is so much faith in doctors and the health system generally. However, the truth of the matter is doctors do not know everything and, as explained already, there is a definite health establishment that has great power. Furthermore, the notion that smoking is incredibly harmful and most smokers will die of lung cancer is so prominent and engrained within us and our health practitioners that the simple truth is lung cancer is often overlooked in non-smokers. The reason for this is simply that doctors are not expecting it to be there, and thus often do not look for it. This is detection bias.

The phrase "there are lies, damn lies, and then there are statistics" probably has no greater relevance than in the field of smoking, and there is no doubt that detection bias leads to misleading and false statistics that only worsen the belief that smoking causes such harm, and this in turn simply increases the chances of detection bias. It is a vicious cycle.

Of course, many people will deny detection bias exists and claim doctors know what they are doing, that this is simply an excuse used by smokers to defend their habit. Whilst there may be logic in this line of reasoning, there is scientific evidence proving detection bias exists, and exists to a degree that it causes misleading statistics.

In 1959 a study was conducted by Heasman and Lipworth[58] in which they surveyed reports from 75 National Health Service (NHS) hospitals. The NHS is the primary care system in Britain, it is funded through taxes and provides free health care; the alternative is private healthcare, whereby people pay extra money for treatment. In these seventy-five hospitals, physicians diagnosed 338 cases of lung cancer, yet pathologists conducting autopsies discovered 417 cases. Oddly enough, despite the physicians diagnosing 338, they diagnosed the same patients as the pathologists only in 227 cases. However, it would appear logical that the pathologists would have a greater ability to determine diseases within the body as they perform autopsies and as such can have the body cut open to see what is really going on inside – an advantage the physicians do not have. This means that if the pathologists were

---

[58] Heasman, M.A., Lipworth, L. (1966) *Accuracy of Certification of Cause of Death*, Studies on Medical and Population Subjects

correct, 111 (33%) of the diagnoses of the attending physicians were false positive, while 190 (46%) genuine cases of lung cancer were overlooked.

Nothing adds validity to a conclusion more than identical results yielded elsewhere. The following study is particularly valuable because it has a different location than the aforementioned and was conducted a quarter of a century later, when medicine and diagnosis had progressed enormously. The study was published in the September 1986 *Archives of Internal Medicine,* and was conducted at the Yale University School of Medicine by Alvan R. Feinstein.[59] Researchers at Yale obtained records on 3,286 adults who had died between 1971 and 1982, and they found that 153 of these patients had died of lung cancer, a discovery made during autopsy. The researchers then obtained the death certificates for those 153 patients to try to find out their smoking habits. Of the 153, there was inadequate smoking information available for thirteen of them so they were rejected from the study – although the researchers reported that of the thirteen, only seven had been diagnosed with having lung cancer, and six had not. Whilst this is a small survey sample, it still means almost 50% went undetected. Of the other 140, there were thirty-seven cases of lung cancer that had not been diagnosed during the victim's lifetime. 57% of these were non-smokers, 30% were moderate smokers, and only 16% were heavy smokers. The researchers conducting the study concluded that a detection bias was present, whereby doctors were willing and always ready to diagnose lung cancer in a smoker, but reluctant to make the diagnosis in a non-smoker:

> The correct diagnosis had not been made during life in 26% of 153 patients with lung cancer found in necropsies performed between 1971 and 1982. The likelihood of a correct antemortem diagnosis showed distinctive gradients in relation to the patients' history and amount of cigarette smoking, symptomatic manifestations, and anatomic extensiveness of the cancers. However, cigarette smoking still exerted a diagnostic effect in patients with similar symptoms and similar degrees of anatomic spread. Furthermore, if a lesion was present, chest films were more likely to be radiologically interpreted as a cancer in smokers.

---

[59] http://archinte.ama-assn.org/cgi/content/abstract/146/9/1695

The results suggest that smokers receive preferential consideration regarding the diagnosis of lung cancer. This detection bias can have adverse scientific consequences in depriving nonsmokers of suitable therapy, in leading to falsely high estimates of the true magnitude of the smoking/lung cancer association, and in distracting etiologic attention from other agents that may cause lung cancer.

A 1988 study, published in the *American Journal of Epidemiology,* also found detection bias when looking at lung cancer. The researchers were Carolyn K. Wells and Alvan R. Feinstein, whose credentials are the Department of Internal Medicine, Yale University School of Medicine; and Departments of Internal Medicine and Epidemiology, Yale University School of Medicine, Veterans Administration Medical Center respectively. They found that lung cancer is often overlooked during life and ante mortem diagnosis is made preferentially in patients with pulmonary symptoms, smokers and men. In other words, many cases of lung cancer are not detected during life, and doctors tend to only find it after death in people they think are most likely to have it. Thus, many people have undetected lung cancer and it is not known about even after death.
Their conclusion stated that:

> Clinically, the results suggest that women and nonsmokers may be deprived of appropriate diagnosis and therapy unless a diagnostic workup for lung cancer is guided mainly by radiographic findings and presenting manifestations. Statistically, detection bias has probably led to an excessively elevated magnitude for the cigarette smoking-lung cancer association and to a falsely low estimate of Incidence[sic] rates in women.[60]

In real terms, this means that smokers and men appear to have higher rates of lung cancer because doctors are actively looking for it in those groups of people. As a result, non-smokers and women appear to have lower incidence rates because the disease is not believed to often affect them. This gives a false portrayal and allows people to believe smokers are more likely to contract lung cancer,

---

[60] http://aje.oxfordjournals.org/cgi/content/abstract/128/5/1016

when in actual fact the researchers state the magnitude of lung cancer in smokers is "excessively elevated".

As with social class, modern results find the same as older results. A 2001 study on detection bias found that it still exists.[61] The purpose of the study was to "examine the possible role of detection bias in the association between amount of cigarette smoking and age at diagnosis of lung cancer." The researchers concluded at the end of their study "detection bias may play a distinctive, although often overlooked, role in the work-up decisions that precede and lead to a diagnosis of lung cancer." Another interesting point they made is that lung cancer often remains undetected during life, meaning in 2001 the same problem existed as it did in 1988: that doctors expect to see lung cancer in cigarette smokers and tend not to look for it in non-smokers. This is a very important point, as it just goes to prove that statistics do not really prove anything. Statistically, smokers suffer lung cancer more than non-smokers. However, this could be due to other factors in the smokers' life, as well as simply that non-smokers are less likely to have their lung cancer diagnosed. The simple fact is that non-smokers also suffer from lung cancer, and just because they statistically do not get it as often as smokers does not mean smoking is the cause in smokers. Of course, anti-smokers deny this and repeat the mantra that lung cancer has only been a problem since smoking became socially acceptable. This is not true at all, and we will look at that now. First, though, it is worth pointing out that people have been smoking tobacco for millennia; it is highly unlikely that in all the time people have been smoking that it has only become a dangerous habit in the past sixty years. Some people will point out that it is only due to medical advances that we know of lung cancer, and this may well be true, but just because we have not been able to diagnose lung cancer for all the time people have been smoking proves nothing – people through the ages would have been able to document specific symptoms, and when the term 'lung cancer' was coined the symptoms displayed would have been identical to those recorded earlier in history. This is, in fact, what happened.

---

[61] http://www.sciencedirect.com/science?
_ob=ArticleURL&_udi=B6T44-42SGGS0-4&_user=10&_rdoc=1&_fmt=&_o
rig=search&_sort=d&view=c&_version=1&_urlVersion=0&_userid=10&md5
=adbf095a27171231942b2a300e2b29a0

An argument exists that lung cancer was a rare disease until the 1930s, when smoking became a prominent activity and lung cancer became a more common disease. It is a well known fact that cancer victims often die as a result of malnutrition or wasting away, and it is essential to remember this. In the first part of the 20th Century any disease which resulted in coughing, wasting away and emaciation was listed under 'consumption', which we now know as tuberculosis. All tuberculosis deaths were included under the heading, and there is no doubt that cancer also was – lung cancer especially causes coughing and often the symptoms of it appear to be problems with the respiratory systems. Funk and Wagnalls 1912 Encyclopaedia says for consumption to look under "pthisis" which it defines as:

> a group of afflictions, but it is generally used to indicate pulmonary consumption i.e. a more or less advancing process of lung destruction, associated with progressive emaciation and other characteristics and symptoms. This is a disease of grave importance, from its frequency and fatal tendency. It has been estimated that consumption is responsible for one-seventh of the mortality of Europe.

The first thing this definition tells us is the symptoms of consumption are very similar or identical to lung cancer, leaving no doubt that any lung cancer deaths would have been listed under consumption. Secondly, it appears consumption was a major cause of death, meaning that there is no basis for the theory that lung cancer was rare until the 1930s. Whilst lung cancer may not have had its own definition, the disease itself was most certainly present before the 1930s. A 1942 editorial in the *British Medical Journal* stated "It is doubtful whether the higher incidence of cancer of the lung observed in recent years is real or only apparent"[62] and offered, amongst factors for an artificial rise, increased diagnosis of the disease. This is the most likely scenario. Indeed, we even know how diagnosis improved and why it was the 1930s specifically that showed more lung cancer cases: mass miniature radiography. This was developed in 1935 and started to be used in Britain in 1936 to screen for tuberculosis;[63] lorries would arrive at school playgrounds

---

[62]Cancer of the lung (editorial) *British Medical Journal* (1942) 1:672-673

[63]http://www.sciencemuseum.org.uk/broughttolife/objects/display.aspx?id=10429

or specific areas within a town, such as a car park, factory yard, or local public health clinic, for people to get screened. Naturally, the people most likely to get screened were those with a cough as that was the most obvious sign of tuberculosis. As one may expect, lung cancer and tuberculosis look entirely different on an x-ray, and the new diagnostic method allowed doctors to not only make a clear distinction between the diseases, but also find numerous new cases of lung cancer that would have previously been overlooked. The scale of this new diagnostic technique cannot be understated. School children had no choice but to be tested; a van would arrive and the pupils would be taken out by class to be x-rayed. For the rest of the population, posters were put up across the country saying where the van would be and when. The fear of tuberculosis was similar to the fear of cancer today; people were scared they would be stricken by the disease and would therefore endeavour to get checked. As previously mentioned, the most obvious symptom of tuberculosis is a dry cough, and the same is true for lung cancer. As such, it was very easy for misdiagnosis to occur prior to mass miniature radiography, and it is similarly clear to see why a sudden surge in lung cancer rates occurred in the 1930s. This decade saw not only a new diagnostic tool, but it being used with extreme efficiency. Prior to this time, diagnosis would have taken place through educated opinion and a doctor using his knowledge of the diseases to make a diagnostic decision. However, with tuberculosis and lung cancer having such similar symptoms, and the former being so prominent in people's minds, it stands to reason that doctors would typically overlook lung cancer. With the advent of mass miniature radiography, such misdiagnosis would have been largely avoided. Furthermore, with the screening van or lorry being so prominent and easily accessible – a conscious decision by the authorities – an increased number of people would have been checked, either compulsorily or voluntarily through fear or increased education. An increase in numbers alone would account for higher cases of both diseases, but the newly-available tool allowed, for the first time ever, a solid way of differentiating victims of tuberculosis and lung cancer.

The Historical Statistics of the United States, published by the Government Printing Office, have cancer statistics from 1900 to 1970. The statistics do not differentiate between different types of cancer, but this is understandable due to the limited understanding of the disease at the time. Below is a table showing the numbers, from the Historical Statistics, of deaths per 100,000 for tuberculosis, cancer and influenza and pneumonia, for the aforementioned time frame.

| Year | Tuberculosis | Cancer | I n f l u e n z a , pneumonia |
|------|--------------|--------|------------------------------|
| 1970 | 2.6 | 162.8 | 30.9 |
| 1960 | 6.1 | 149.2 | 37.3 |
| 1950 | 22.5 | 139.8 | 31.3 |
| 1940 | 45.9 | 120.3 | 70.3 |
| 1930 | 71.1 | 97.4 | 102.5 |
| 1920 | 113.1 | 83.4 | 207.3 |
| 1910 | 153.8 | 76.2 | 155.9 |
| 1900 | 194.4 | 64.0 | 202.2 |

An instantly apparent feature is that there is a very neat, linear inverse relation between the cancer figures and the tuberculosis figures – as the years went on, the tuberculosis figures decrease considerably, whilst the cancer figures increase considerably. It becomes clear, then, that cancer – if not all of them then certainly of the lung – was listed under consumption before being recognised as a disease itself.

With time, diagnosis continued to improve. In the 1940s and 1950s physicians had the aid of bronchoscopes, and after the war antibiotics allowed them to discover an underlying cancer in patients previously thought to be suffering from pneumonia. It is without doubt that the 1930s saw a huge leap in medical understanding, and this was reflected in the increasing lung cancer rates. It stands to reason that as such advancements were made diagnosis would improve and, as the table demonstrates, there was not actually much of a rise in lung disease *per se*, but rather a decrease in tuberculosis and a rise in cancer. This fits perfectly with the suggestion that improved measures, such as mass miniature radiography, forced numerous cases of lung diseases cases to be recognised as cancer rather than tuberculosis.

Thus, it is apparent that lung cancer was *not* a rare disease until the 1930s; it was just often misdiagnosed as tuberculosis and as science progressed this discrepancy was revealed.

## Chapter 5: Smoking and Cancer

Cancer is undoubtedly the largest health concern of smoking. The public is led to believe that smoking is the single biggest preventable cause of the disease and that a large proportion of smokers will die from it. Not so readily admitted is that a similar proportion of non-smokers will probably contract cancer too, if not more. As mentioned in the Introduction, Cancer Research UK state that roughly a third of cancer occurs in smokers – meaning that approximately two-thirds occurs in non-smokers.

There is a large body of work to show that smoking causes cancer. Cancer Research UK states that "In the UK, smoking kills five times more people than road accidents, overdoses, murder, suicide and HIV all put together." and "Smoking and passive smoking cause nine out of ten lung cancers."[64] Of course, no reference or citation is given for either statement.

Before going any further I would like to include an excerpt from an article written by Dr Siepmann, M.D. writing for the *Journal of Theoretics*.[65]

> smoking does not cause lung cancer. It is only one of many risk factors for lung cancer. I initially was going to write an article on how the professional literature and publications misuse the language by saying "smoking causes lung cancer", but the more that I looked into how biased the literature, professional organizations [sic], and the media are, I modified this article to one on trying to put the relationship between smoking and cancer into perspective.

Dr Siepmann makes a point that many forget: 'cause' and 'factor' are different things. For example, striking a match and putting it to paper will cause a fire; a cause is a sequence of events that will lead to a definite outcome. A factor, on the other hand, is when an action *may possibly* cause an outcome.

Regarding the studies showing smoking causes cancer, two things need to be addressed. Firstly, at what point can we be sure something is a causative agent, and secondly, how objective are

---

[64] http://info.cancerresearchuk.org/healthyliving/smokingandtobacco/?a=5441

[65] http://www.journaloftheoretics.com/Editorials/Vol-1/e1-4.htm

these studies? Regarding the former, what exactly is 'cause'? Surely it means that a factor, or myriad of factors, have undisputedly caused the onset of something. This is not the same as a statistical correlation. Really and truly, if smoking *causes* illness and disease, given the millions of smokers worldwide both now and in the past there would be an epidemic of such illnesses. Furthermore, the rates of smoking have been declining in America and the UK since the 1960s, yet illnesses have not decreased accordingly – cancer rates have skyrocketed. The only way we can say smoking causes cancer is when all other factors have been eradicated, and this has not yet been done in a human study. For example, it is all well and good to show a statistical link between smokers and cancer, but what is often overlooked are other factors such as stress, diet, sleeping patterns, healthcare, and lifestyles. Smokers, for instance, are less likely to follow a healthy lifestyle than non-smokers. Most cigarette smokers come from lower social classes meaning they have poorer diets and healthcare than non-smokers, are more likely to have more stressful jobs requiring long hours of physical labour, and generally have a less relaxed lifestyle.

All these things apparently increase the risk of cancer, so how can tobacco products be singled out? Quite simply, they cannot. As a matter of fact, the only studies conducted where smoking is the only single factor are the animal studies, and these have failed to conclusively link smoking with lung cancer. With regards to human studies, the only true way smoking could be shown to induce cancer would be to get a group of children, all with the same medical history in their families, split them into two groups, one with smokers and one without, expose them to the same lifestyles, including diet, healthcare plans, jobs and so on, and follow them throughout their lives. Clearly, this is impossible.

In the recent court case *Mrs Margaret McTear vs. Imperial Tobacco Limited*, Lord Nimmo Smith, in his conclusion of the trial, stated the following:

> I must base my decisions about questions of fact on the evidence, and that alone.
>
> It is not within judicial knowledge that cigarette smoking can cause lung cancer: this is an issue which I am duty-bound to approach with an open mind and to decide on the basis of the evidence led before me; and the burden of proving it is on the pursuer.

In any event, the pursuer has failed to prove individual causation. Epidemiology cannot be used to establish causation in any individual case, and the use of statistics applicable to the general population to determine the likelihood of causation in an individual is fallacious. Given that there are possible causes of lung cancer other than cigarette smoking, and given that lung cancer can occur in a non-smoker, it is not possible to determine in any individual case whether but for an individual's cigarette smoking he probably would not have contracted lung cancer.[66]

What he is saying then, is that there is no evidence to confidently say that smoking causes lung cancer, at least not on an individual level. That is to say that even if the evidence that smoking may cause cancer is convincing, that is no reason to suggest or to believe that any individual cancer cases in smokers are caused by smoking. Since non-smokers can also contract the disease we cannot be sure that the cancers in smokers would not have occurred had they not smoked. It is very important to note that the link between smoking and cancer is a statistical one, not a scientific one. There is no scientific evidence to show that smoking causes cancer, there are only statistics which, as everyone knows, can be used to prove whatever the researcher wants them to. We can never be sure whether a diagnosed case of lung cancer is indeed lung cancer unless an autopsy is conducted, and comparatively few autopsies actually take place. This goes back to the detection bias point: doctors are quick to diagnose lung cancer in smokers, but more reluctant in non-smokers. As the studies have shown, detection bias is a very real problem and unless autopsies are conducted on all deceased people (not just those diagnosed with the disease) then we cannot be sure the diagnosis was right. In other words, the notion that smokers suffer more lung cancer is highly unlikely to be true. Even if one were to reject the above point on autopsies, the chapter on detection bias should serve as proof that not all cases are as they seem.

Furthermore, an excerpt from *Smoking. Psychology and Pharmacology* states:

---

[66] http://www.scotcourts.gov.uk/opinions/2005CSOH69.html

The statistical association between smoking and diseases such as lung cancer could arise because smoking is an aggravating factor or a cause of such diseases; this is a conclusion which is widely accepted. However, many people, not exclusively in the tobacco industry, have argued against this view (e.g. Fisher 1958; Burch 1974; Eysenck 1965). A correlation between smoking and disease does not itself prove a causal connection. It remains possible that other variables, present more frequently or more strongly in smokers than in non-smokers, underlie both the smoking and the disease.[67]

Thus, despite the widespread opinion that smoking definitely causes cancer and no person in their right mind would question or challenge this notion, there are in fact researchers and scientists who do challenge it. They also point out other reasons which explain the statistical link between smoking and lung cancer.

It is relevant here to mention a study showing that, if there is indeed a risk to smoking, it has been grossly exaggerated. The study in question was reported in the *Associated Press*, May 23rd 1995, and was conducted by Dr. Gary Strauss. The study consisted of Strauss analysing 685 lung cancer patients at Brigham and Women's hospital in Boston between 1988 and 1994. Strauss found that 59% of the patients were non-smokers when their cancers were diagnosed; 8% of these had never smoked, and 51% had given up at some point. Of the 51% who had given up, almost a quarter had stopped smoking over twenty years previously and the average time of stopping was six years. So, almost 60% of the cancer victims were non-smokers, and stopping smoking did not prevent them getting cancer.

Dr David Burns, of the University of California, points out in the same article that giving up smoking is no by means a safe guard against cancer, and says:

---

[67] Ashton, H; Stepney, R. (1982) *Smoking Psychology and Pharmacology* Tavistock Publications (p 127)

These folks have done what we told them to do, yet they are still at substantially increased risk. What can we do for them? We owe these people an answer.

The truth is out. The respective organisations have been so concerned with demonising tobacco and smoking that very little else is said about cancer and how we can help prevent it. Burns suggested that it could be possible to have a genetic test to spot lung cancer, and whilst this is a good idea it is not by any means the only, or ultimate, way of protecting oneself from cancer. Genetics will be looked at later in this chapter as it is a very interesting notion with regards to illness and disease, but at the same time it is important to remember that it is not the only factor.

Before examining the studies linking smoking with cancer, two things need to be considered:

Firstly, there are three terms to bear in mind: validity, reliability and generality. Validity determines how well a study relates to real life. Reliability determines how well a study can be replicated; typically a study with high validity will have low reliability and vice versa. This is because reliable results typically come from laboratory studies using strict controls that have little bearing on the real world. Generality determines how well results can be applied universally.

Secondly, as mentioned in the Introduction, within the health establishment exist agendas, such as allowing government members to increase the size and power of their agencies and further their careers. Studies are conducted to fulfil these agendas; consequently, results are not always as they seem. Therefore, the studies themselves must be carefully looked at as well as the results to see what controls were included, what were left out, and what effect this may have had.

## Animal Studies

When trying to determine if a substance is harmful or safe for human consumption animals are almost always used in experiments to see how the substance affects them. Rodents are actually fairly similar to humans and animal studies are an effective and reliable way of testing how a product will affect humans. Using animals is a mainstay of real science and, whatever one's stance on the ethics of animal testing, it is unsurpassable as an initial screening test of a substance. Since countless numbers of animals can be used, from a variety of species, scientists can gather if a product is harmful to any or all, and in what form and at what dose, etc.

There have been many animal studies involving tobacco, which is no surprise. What will be surprising to many, though, is the fact that no researcher has ever managed to induce lung cancer in an animal with tobacco products. To clarify, this does not mean that no animal has contracted lung cancer in a study, but the figures of animals who did get the disease was so low that it is not possible to claim smoking caused it. Given this, it is a wonder so many people – especially those in high places – succumb to the belief that smoking, or tobacco in any form, is deadly to humans. After all, how can a product be essentially harmless to every species of animal tested (which is an extensive list) but be so harmful to human beings? Apparently we are the only species that are intolerant to tobacco, which is a ridiculous notion.

Animals have been used in smoking studies for decades, and were mentioned in the 1964 Surgeon General's Report. Movietone News, an old newsreel company, had a film on smoking beagles which was shot during the 1950s or 1960s. The study had the beagles strapped to a long bench, side-by-side, with face masks. The masks forced them to smoke lit cigarettes as a device would light a cigarette each time one was finished. Therefore, the beagles were forced to smoke continuously; something that not even the most hardened smoker does, so the study is not at all realistic.

Whilst it is not known for certain if it is these specific beagles that the Surgeon General mentioned in the 1964 Report, the claim was made, in the Report, that the dogs were not inhaling deeply. Whilst this is irrelevant, given that if smoke is entering the lungs then it is entering the lungs, how deep it goes is inconsequential, the video footage from Movietone News appears to show the beagles inhaling very deeply.

In the 1964 Report the Surgeon General admitted that none of the animal studies had succeeded in inducing lung cancer, with the "possible exception of dogs". Nonetheless, in the 1971 Report the Surgeon General admits that the experiments with dogs, using smoking machines as in the original study, had failed. The 1971 Report also describes a new experiment which was conducted by a government physician, Oscar Auerbach, and others. In this study the Beagles were forced to smoke in a "more natural" way. The study consisted of eighty-six Beagles having their throats slit and tracheotomy tubes inserted. Apparently the dogs had been trained to smoke cigarettes using the tracheotomies. The methods of this study are not remotely natural, given that no person smokes in those manners.

The results were shown in a table, showing the number of dogs that survived for two and a half years. The dogs were also in three groups: those smoking regular cigarettes, those smoking filtered cigarettes, and those not smoking. Of the eighty-six, seventy-eight smoked and eight did not. Of the eight controls who did not smoke none of the Beagles died, and of the smoking dogs there were twenty-four deaths but not from cancer. There were various causes, such as "aspiration of food" and lung fibrosis (this is a condition where the alveoli become chronically inflamed and fibrous tissue builds up as the lung tries to heal itself. In the majority of cases the cause is unknown, although inhaling asbestos, ground stone or metal dust can cause it. However, smoking appears

to be entirely innocent). Despite there being no lung cancers to report, Auerbach did claim that two of the dogs from the non-filter cigarette group developed early invasive squamous cell carcinoma in the bronchi. It is interesting to note that no adjustments appear to have been made for stress levels. The dogs were forced to wear 'smoking masks' and inhale thirty cigarettes a day, their heads locked in place by two boards, and when they were not in these contraptions they were in small kennels.[68] It is not surprising they became ill! What is also interesting is that a PBS document supposedly exposing tobacco companies knew cigarettes caused lung cancer, based on Auerbach's experiment, actually shows "only one in ten heavy smokers get lung cancer".[69] The tobacco industry paper actually states that Auerbach's study appears to be conclusive in showing dog's develop cancer from smoking and this may translate to humans, but not definitely. It also states that "there are certain short-comings of the experiment and it is easier to see these in hind-sight". Indeed, and one huge short-coming is the fact there were only eight non-smoking dogs!

---

[68] http://www.acigawis.co.uk/smoking_beagles_at_ici.htm

[69] http://www.pbs.org/wgbh/pages/frontline/shows/settlement/case/dogs.html

When results have only been obtained from one study scientists warn to approach it with caution, as it could be the result of bias, fraud, or just fluke. The 1982 Report has the Surgeon General describing the experiment again but remarking that the "observation has not been repeated so far". In other words, either the study has not been re-done or the results have not shown smoking to be harmful to the dogs. Of course, one major problem with the study is that it only has eight non-smoking dogs – hardly a valid measure when there were seventy-eight dogs forced to smoke. For all we know, if there had been seventy-eight controls then there could have been more deaths than the study group. The fact that the observation had not been repeated in 1982 (and still has not in 2009) may indicate that the Surgeon General is politely saying that the study might have been fraudulent. Furthermore, the Surgeon General declines to divulge any more information explaining in what way the observation has not been repeated – for instance, whether the dogs were all fine, or whether the study was never conducted again. The fact that the Surgeon General decides to keep this to himself leads me to the conclusion that there is something to hide, but maybe I am just cynical.

The 1982 Report appears to have the Surgeon General trying desperately to explain why animals were not developing cancer from smoking, and on page 185 we are told that one major problem is that the animals are unwilling to inhale:

> Furthermore, laboratory animals are not willing to inhale aerosols very deeply and are especially reluctant to inhale tobacco smoke. Inhalation studies have been explored by training Rhesus monkeys and baboons to smoke cigarettes. This approach does not produce respiratory neoplasms because of insufficient exposure time and because of the tendency of the animals merely to puff rather than to inhale.

Apparently the Surgeon General had forgotten the 1964 Report, in which it is written that animals did not inhale *deeply* – in 1982 we are being told they do not inhale at all. Plus, of course, the video footage showed to anyone who wished to view it that, actually, the animals did inhale.

On page 175 we are given some telling information:

> For inhalation tests of the carcinogenicity of tobacco smoke and various fractions of tobacco smoke, hamsters are preferable to rats and mice because they respond with a higher incidence of airway tumors

This is a blatant occurrence of bias: they used animals they knew were more susceptible to tumours of the places that smoke will make contact. So, despite them being likely to contract diseases anyway, the researchers will be able to blame it on smoking. We are also given an insight into how unrealistic the methods used are:

> In lieu of using large inhalation chambers in which animals are exposed, it is possible to use chambers into which the head and nose of individual animals are fitted. The test material is then forced into the chamber, resulting in an inhalation exposure. Relatively few animals can be treated with a given chamber by this method, however.

This is a completely ridiculous way to test the toxicity of tobacco smoke, for two reasons. Firstly, no person is contained in a smoke filled chamber. Ever. Secondly, any animal being used has a much smaller lung capacity and airways than humans, and thus the effect on them will be far worse than on us. That being said, the fact that none of these animals contracted lung cancer from smoke goes to show how harmful it really is.

Page 185 appears to be the page on which the Surgeon General reveals how useless the experiments are, and on this page and the following page he describes failed experiments with Golden hamsters. About halfway down page 185, though, we are told of an experiment that succeeded in causing tumours of the respiratory tract in rats, thanks to a new "advanced inhalation device". The Surgeon General writes of a 1980 experiment in which:

> investigators at the Oak Ridge National Laboratory succeeded in obtaining tumors of the respiratory-tract of rats using a highly developed smoke inhalation device (43, 126). On 5 days each week over their entire lifespan, 80 rats were exposed to air-diluted smoke (10 percent) of seven cigarettes (one cigarette per hour). At the end of the experiment, a large number of rats had developed hyperplasia or metaplasia in the epithelium of the nasal system, the larynx, or the trachea. Seven of the eighty

smoke-exposed rats had tumors of the respiratory tract, including five animals with pulmonary adenomas, two with alveologenic carcinomas, one with a squamous carcinoma of the lung, and one with adenocarcinoma and squamous cell carcinoma in the nasal cavity. One alveologenic carcinoma was observed in 30 sham-exposed control rats; no respiratory tract tumors were seen in 63 untreated control rats.

To put this into perspective: of eighty rats, seven developed tumours of the respiratory tract, one developed a squamous carcinoma of the lung, and one adenocarcinoma and squamous cell carcinoma in the nasal cavity. So only one of them developed lung cancer, which is certainly not enough to conclude the tobacco caused it.

It is worth looking at the new "advanced inhalation device" mentioned, as it is only since this was developed that the tumours actually occurred. The device is the MaddoxORNL smoking machine, and is referred to in an article by A.P. Wehner et al in *Toxicology and Applied Pharmacology* in 1981 on pages 1-17 where the authors describe an experiment involving eighty female rats. The rats were forced to inhale eight cigarettes a day for two years. Of the eighty, one developed a carcinoma.

First things first, rats are prone to tumours. The two most common causes of death to domestic rats are tumours and respiratory illness. Secondly, rats have an average lifespan of two years. So even if these rats were forced to inhale smoke from the minute they were born, they were smoking as much as some humans for most of their life. They were certainly elderly at the end of the experiment, and yet only one rat developed a carcinoma. For seventy nine rats to reach over two years and not develop tumours is not far off miraculous, so for anyone to claim the smoking machine is the reason that one tumour developed is simply not true. If it were, then why did the other seventy-nine not get tumours? Another very important point is one touched on earlier; that the size difference between rats and humans cannot be overstated. For rats to consume eight cigarettes a day – which is the same general quantity as many humans – for essentially their whole lives is quite amazing. Rats are prone to respiratory problems, they have very sensitive airways and the size of their nasal passage, throat and lungs is tiny, especially when compared to humans. Given this, it is more than a little strange that rats, who weigh between 200-800 grams, can go through their life unaffected by heavy smoking, but there is apparently no safe limit of even second-hand smoke for people.

Something else that is very strange is that there appears to be no additional animal experiments (with rats or other animals) since 1980 which replicate the above. This is perplexing because that is the year that the advanced machine was used, apparently with success (though not quite), yet it was not followed up. It begs the question of 'why not?', after all, one would expect for researchers, whether they are objectively researching the effects of tobacco or setting out to prove smoking is harmful, to follow up such results to see if they were consistent or a fluke. It is my suspicion that such studies were conducted but not reported because they failed. I could be wrong, of course, but there is really no other explanation, other than they were not repeated at all. And if this the case, it still begs the same question, because there is no way the researchers – or other researchers – would feel content with the results of one small study. Rather, they would want to repeat it in an attempt to prove without question that smoking is harmful. After all, showing nine out of eighty rats can develop tumours, one of eighty sham-exposed rats can get a lung carcinoma, and one out of eighty rats forced to smoke for two years is not nearly conclusive evidence – besides all being incredibly small numbers, they are also from single studies.

There are, though, other studies. An article in *Toxicology and Applied Pharmacology* in 1989 described an experiment where male and female rats were forced to inhale high concentrations of cigarette smoke for a period of twenty-two weeks, or five and a half months. After that period, the rats were killed and there were investigations to see the effect the smoke had had on the DNA adducts. It was concluded that "inhaled cigarette smoke induces lung DNA adducts which may play an important role in cigarette-induced lung carcinogenesis". Apparently, though, none of their study rats developed any tumours. If they had, we surely would have been told of it.

Another study on rats appeared in 1985 in the journal *Cancer Research*. However, as with the aforementioned study, the researchers do not mention any harm to the rats as a result of smoke. All that is said is that the smoke reduced the production level of cytotoxin, a substance that is thought to be toxic to certain types of tumour cells. In other words, cigarette smoke reduces (not eliminates) the production level of a substance that is thought to, but not proven to, be toxic to certain types, but not all types, of tumour cells. The only logical answer to this is 'so what?' it is not a substance the rats need, the smoke does not get rid of it, and the smoke caused no harm. In other words, another animal study failed.

In addition to the above, a 1985 report from the Microbiological Laboratory at Bethesda mentioned a critical study. An investigation was carried out over nine years and with over 10,000 mice, specially bred to contract lung cancer, which were forced to inhale cigarette smoke. The results are very telling indeed: not one of the mice, developed squamous cell carcinoma, which is the type of lung cancer that is said to be caused by tobacco smoking. Of course, of the ten thousand mice some did develop various types of cancer, but the incidence was the same as the non-smoking control group. That is a very interesting find: 10,000 mice, some developed cancers, but none developed the 'smoker's' lung cancer.

One study that proves unsurpassable actually goes so far as to show that smoking may *prevent* lung cancer. The study in question was not actually planned. The truth is that every animal, without exception, that has been exposed to radioactive particles has contracted lung cancer and died. In any animal study, the animals are used in that study and then destroyed to prevent 'cross-contamination' i.e. to prevent unwanted or unknown variables affecting results. On one occasion, a few thousand mice from a smoking study somehow found their way into the radioactive particle experiment (whether it was accidental or the researchers knew what really caused lung cancer, I do not know) and, unlike the thousands before them, 60% of the smoking group survived. The only variable was that they had been exposed to tobacco smoke.[70] A possible explanation is that the mucous production that smoking stimulates formed a protective lining on the lungs, thus preventing radioactive particles penetrating the lung tissue.

---

[70] http://tobaccodocuments.org/landman/507927406-7466.html?
zoom=750&ocr_position=above_foramatted&start_page=11

There are further animal studies which suggest smoking protects against lung cancer. One such study, entitled *Inhalation Bioassay of Cigarette Smoke in Rats*,[71] found that:

> the highest number of tumors [sic] occurred in the untreated control [non-smoking] rats. The next highest number of tumors [sic] occurred in rats subject to sham smoking, i.e. rats which were placed in the smoking machine without smoke exposure, and the lowest number of tumors [sic] occurred in the smoke-exposed rats. Among the latter, the largest number of tumors [sic] occurred in rats exposed to smoke from cigarettes having the lowest level of nicotine.

Further to this, Professors Mori and Sakai of Tokyo University stated in *Cancer*, April 1984, that there was an increase in lung cancer in non-smokers and this increase was in fact higher than smokers. Also, in studies where dogs are exposed to uranium ore dust they all (100%) contracted lung cancer. However, Cross et al reported in *Health Physics* (42:32 1982) that their research showed that if the dogs inhaled tobacco smoke at the same time the rate of lung cancer was greatly reduced. This is very important, as if there is a constant rate of 100% of lung cancer in dogs exposed to uranium ore dust and this is greatly reduced with exposure to tobacco smoke then there is no arguing the tobacco smoke, for whatever reason, is protecting the dogs from developing cancer.

Professor Schrauzer, President of the International Association of Bio-inorganic Chemists, actually testified before a United States congressional committee in 1982 that scientists had known for a long that there were certain constituents of tobacco smoke that act as anti-carcinogens (they work to prevent cancer, as opposed to carcinogens which cause it) in test animals. He went on to say that when known carcinogens are applied to the animals the application of constituents of cigarette smoke counter them. He continued further, testifying on oath to the committee, that "no ingredient of cigarette smoke has been shown to cause human lung cancer" and "no-one has been able to produce lung cancer in laboratory animals from smoking."

---

[71] A.P. Wehrner, et al. (1981) *Inhalation Bioassy of Cigarette Smoke in Rats* Journal of Toxiology & Applied Pharmacology, Vol. 61: pp 1-17

On the 13th January 1995 the *Wall Street Journal* reported a study involving animals that was partly funded by the U.S. National Institutes of Health. The report stated that a researcher from Buffalo, named John Pauly, was studying some tissue from a lung cancer victim who was a smoker, and he found a tiny particle of cellulose acetate, which is a part of a cigarette filter. From this, Pauly hypothesised that pieces of cigarette filters detach from the cigarette and become embedded in the lungs and cause lung cancer, and he then conducted an experiment with mice to see if he was right. The experiment consisted of Pauly putting tiny pieces of filters, coated with cigarette tar, in the lungs of six mice. This is interesting given that there is still no common consensus on what cigarette tar actually is. Six months later, when he opened them up, he found the particles still in the lungs and concluded that he was right: pieces of cigarette filters get in the lungs of smokers, stay there, and cause cancer. He overlooked just one little problem, though: none of the mice had cancer. All he really proved was that the pieces of filter stayed in the lungs, nothing more.

Predictably, with the rise of the second-hand smoke idea there have been machines developed that subject rats to second-hand smoke, instead of making them actively smoke. These started in the early 1990s and in the May 28th 1994 issue of *The Los Angeles Times* Sheryl Stolberg wrote about experiments that had been going on since 1991 in which rats were exposed to continuous concentrations of smoke up to 4,000 micrograms per cubic metre. Chapter six goes into detail of what the actual concentrations are for humans in public places, but even bar workers are not exposed to *continuous* smoke, which, besides ridiculously high levels of smoke, renders these studies completely unrealistic. However, despite the excessively high concentrations of smoke administered to animals that are far smaller than humans, each study concluded that no significant harm came to the animals. The only exception was one researcher named Davis at UC claiming to have found a 6% reduction in birth weight of baby rats from the exposed parents.

Given that 'regular' animals failed to highlight smoking as deadly, researchers developed animals genetically susceptible to cancer. After the failed attempts with 'regular' animals, and the fact that sponsors did not want such results, researchers decided to take drastic measures. A recent study, conducted on behalf on Pfizer in

2004,[72] used F334 rats to try to prove smoking causes cancer. F334 rats are genetically bred to develop various cancers and have a lifespan of 24 months. A/J mice are the same – genetically bred to develop cancer and have a shortened lifespan. These breeds of rodents have been used for many years, as evidenced previously with the Surgeon General quote referring to the Golden Hamsters. The aim is, evidently, to expose genetically doomed animals to tobacco smoke so the researchers can then falsely claim that the smoke was responsible. A further benefit to the researchers is that because such animals develop cancers all over their body the cancerous cells compete for blood and nutrients – resulting in larger and more numerous cancerous tumours at the site with most nutrient-rich blood.

Numerous studies have shown that nicotine stimulates vascular growth [73] [74] [75]and, as such, when cancer exists in an organism it will migrate to the site of the body where it is more likely to survive. Nonetheless, despite the rats in the study having higher incidences of lung cancers (which was no surprise given the aforementioned), the rats still proved a medicinal property of tobacco smoke: the 'low exposure' group outlived the non-smoking rats. The 'low-exposure' group had 100 mg of smoke particles per cubic metre, or the equivalent of ten full-strength cigarettes every five minutes, in a one cubic metre box, six hours a day, five days a week for thirty months. Thirty months is actually six months longer than the F334 rat's life-expectancy. The 'high exposure' group, however, were forced to inhale so much smoke that some were physically asphyxiated. In fact, it has long been known that smoke-exposed animals outlive animals not exposed to tobacco smoke, with one example coming from a 1979 study:

> The increased incidences in the smoke-exposed hamsters were not necessarily caused by the smoke exposures, but

---

[72] http://toxsci.oxfordjournals.org/cgi/content/full/81/2/280

[73] http://ajp.amjpathol.org/cgi/content/abstract/160/2/413

[74] http://www3.interscience.wiley.com/journal/104541376/abstract

[75] http://jap.physiology.org/cgi/content/abstract/84/6/2089

might be explained by the **significantly longer life-span of the smoke-exposed hamsters** [emphasis mine] [76]

The final word on animal studies attempting to produce lung cancer in laboratory animals should come from the 1998 court case of the State of Minnesota suing the tobacco companies for healthcare costs to the State as a result of smoking. There were a number of trial sessions, which saw experts for both the State and the tobacco companies agree that every animal study had failed to induce lung cancer in animals despite numerous attempts with countless animals and at various quantities and concentrations.

The bottom line is this: researchers have tried incredibly hard to produce lung cancer in animals via smoking, yet failed every time. Numerous studies, in the Surgeon General's Reports also, use tricky language to deceive people into thinking cancer has been induced with tobacco smoke, however a thorough read shows that they used condensates of various chemicals found within tobacco smoke to cause skin cancer, which they then blamed on tobacco smoke. However, a condensate is not the same as the same chemical in a tobacco product, and skin cancer can be induced by putting any irritant on an animal, especially bald mice. The Minnesota court case showed, conclusively, that no matter what language is used or tricks are used, no animal study has managed to induce lung cancer via smoking – if it had, the Minnesota lawyers would have shown as much, but not only did they not do that, they admitted the studies had failed. The anti-smoking crusaders hate the animal studies and avoid mentioning them. The ones who do mention them say they were successful and decline to elaborate or explain how they were successful – simply because they were not.

This brings us full circle to what was said at the beginning of the chapter: animals are used to test products to see how harmful they are to humans. When the product fails to harm an animal, it is considered harmless to people. Tobacco appears to be a standalone exception.

## Human Studies

Richard Doll

---

[76] Wehrner A.P. (1979) *Inhalation Studies with Syrian Golden Hamsters* used in http://www2.tobaccodocuments.org/nysa_ti_m2/TI03931992.pdf p.98

Sir Richard Doll was responsible for one of the initial main studies linking smoking with cancer, which is still considered by Cancer Research UK as the ultimate smoking study. Before we look at this study itself there is something very important to address, which quite simply underlines the massive bias and political agendas present regarding smoking studies.

In 2006 Sarah Boseley, health editor of the *Guardian* newspaper, wrote an article explaining that Richard Doll had been paid by chemical companies for 20 years. Monsanto were paying Sir Richard a consultancy fee of $1,500 a day in the mid-1980s, and he also received

> £15,000 fee by the Chemical Manufacturers Association and two other major companies, Dow Chemicals and ICI, for a review that largely cleared vinyl chloride, used in plastics, of any link with cancers apart from liver cancer – a conclusion with which the World Health Organisation disagrees. Sir Richard's review was used by the manufacturers' trade association to defend the chemical for more than a decade.[77]

Further to this, whilst being paid by Monsanto, Doll wrote to a royal Australian commission investigating the potential cancer-causing properties of Agent Orange to say there was no evidence that the chemical caused cancer. Agent Orange was made by Monsanto and was being used by America in the Vietnam War. In other words: Sir Richard Doll was being paid a vast sum of money by chemical manufacturers to cover up evidence that their products caused cancer, and we trust the validity of his work. The politics at work are very clear to see.

Additionally, writing in the December 2001 issue of the *British Medical Journal*, Doll wrote that the study was "devised by Sir Austin Bradford Hill to achieve maximum publicity for the critical link between smoking and lung cancer". What this means, then, is that they did not set out to conduct a serious scientific study into the effects of smoking; they went out with the intention of creating propaganda. This has been ignored by the medical community, but the truth is the truth. In this instance the truth is that Sir Richard Doll, long-revered and respected icon in the anti-smoking field,

---

[77] http://www.guardian.co.uk/science/2006/dec/08/smoking.frontpagenews

created nothing but propaganda and later was paid huge sums of money by chemical manufacturing companies, before even admitting that his studies were worthless.

Doll conducted a study in 1950 with Professor Austin Bradford Hill of the Medical Research Council. It shows a recurring theme, that statistically smokers are more likely to develop lung cancer than non-smokers, without showing an actual causative effect. The study was based on a survey of lung cancer patients in twenty London hospitals and found that smoking was the only factor overwhelmingly implicated in lung cancer and that it was rare for non-smokers to suffer from the disease. At first, though, many greeted the connection between smoking and cancer with scepticism. Smoking was seen as just too 'normal' an activity to be so dangerous. It took seven years for the Ministry of Health to take Doll's findings seriously and even in 1958 one Harley Street physician objected to the Medical Research Council's link between smoking and cancer as "a staggering and most unscientific claim". He went on: "They will be blaming mother's milk next."[78]

The study has such serious flaws it is surprising it ever managed to get published in a medical journal. Firstly, it only looks at London hospitals and not hospitals around the country. London itself is a busy city, full of pollution and, in the 1950s, was full of working-class men working in factories, warehouses and other such dangerous places, so maybe this study simply reinforces the hypothesis that those from the lower classes are more likely to contract lung cancer. To simply look at lung cancer patients and ask if they smoke is not science. In the 1950s 82% of British men smoked – so of course the overwhelming majority of lung cancer patients smoked – so, too, did the overwhelming majority of those without lung cancer. In fact, table four of the study shows that in the lung cancer study group there were two non-smokers and 647 smokers, with twenty-seven non-smokers and 622 smokers in the group without lung cancer. In other words, 99.7% of the entire study were smokers. Such figures do not lend themselves to objectivity or meaningful results: whatever the outcome, the majority would have been smokers. Furthermore, this study does nothing to explore the social status of the lung cancer patients, and has simply isolated smoking as the causative agent of lung cancer

---

[78] http://www.telegraph.co.uk/news/obituaries/1494745/Professor-Sir-Richard-Doll.html

without looking at other possibilities such as air pollution and general lifestyle. Perhaps looking at hospitals in more rural areas would have shown different results.

It is most probable that at this stage of his career Doll was a serious researcher. Rather than intentionally misleading people with this study, it is more likely he was genuinely convinced by his research; he did in fact stop smoking during this study. It may also be that Doll had started to take the view that smoking caused lung cancer many years earlier as he had access to the Nazi research. A 1939 study from Muller is cited among the references of this London Hospital's study so it is evident he had read the investigation and was swayed, at least somewhat, by it. It is entirely possible, then, that Doll believed smoking caused cancer but because of the research's ties to Nazism decided to repeat them, resulting in his suspicions becoming convictions.

Whilst Doll claimed the disease was rare in non-smokers, nowadays we know that non-smokers are often diagnosed with lung cancer, despite the rate of smoking decreasing. It is also true that a very small percentage of smokers contract the disease, nowadays only 5-10% of smokers contract it and that rate was similar or lower in the 1950s. It is evident, therefore, that something else needs to be considered, and Doll did not consider it. For a study like this to ever be valid it needs to have a larger sample with hospitals from different areas. This would account for the different lifestyles not only of the social classes but also those in the city and the countryside, as well as accounting for the difference in air pollution. It would also need to look at the lifestyle of individual patients rather than merely asking whether they smoked or not. Finally, it would need to obtain a large sample from people without lung cancer to see whether or not they smoked. As stated already, 82% of British men smoked in the 1950s and so it stands to reason that most people in hospital at the time would have smoked – but so would those outside the hospital. This is no different to asking if the people drank coffee or ate white bread – it is nothing but a conversation starter and has no scientific merit. Doll's recollections of the study are somewhat interesting:

> By the time we had data on several hundred patients it was obvious that the principal difference between the patients with and without lung cancer was their smoking habits, and we had to make up our minds whether the association was

due to chance, bias, confounding, or to cause and effect. The evidence that led us to conclude that it was due to the last (and which led me to give up smoking in 1949) is described in our first paper.

Actually it is not "obvious" at all, as almost 96% of the control group were smokers. Therefore, it was not an isolated factor.

Now we will look at Doll's most famous study in detail. The study was a prospective study and was conducted in 1956 by Doll and Hill. The study involved a questionnaire sent out to all members of the medical profession in the UK. The first problem with this is that all results are dependent on doctors responding, and not all doctors asked to participate actually did. Questionnaires have a self-selected response and therefore any statistics and percentages are going to be flawed – after all, saying, for example, that 60% of doctors smoke means that 60% of the respondent participants smoke, and if only 50% responded then that 60% is a grossly misleading number.

Another major discrepancy with the study is that all the deaths in which lung cancer was a contributing cause were classified as deaths from lung cancer, even though the direct cause of death may have been something else.[79]

In 1976, Doll issued a paper reporting that daily cigarette consumption by the British doctors had declined from 9.1 in 1951 to 3.6 in 1971. Doll then claimed that a direct consequence of this was a 38% reduction in lung cancer death rates amongst the doctors.

However, in a 1978 paper[80] Philip R. J. Burch, a professor of Medical Physics at the University of Leeds (a non-smoker, whose principal life work was an attempt to develop a unified theory of cancer), showed that Doll had simply compared the lung cancer death rates among the doctors with the lung cancer death rates for the entire British male population. Accordingly, Burch re-plotted the data to compare the doctors with other doctors and showed that actually the risk for lung cancer amongst doctors had increased by 31%. While Doll released results showing that

---

[79] Surgeon General Report, 1964, page 101

[80] Burch, P; (1978) *Smoking and Lung Cancer: the Problem of Inferring Cause* J. Royal Statistical Society

stopping smoking had reduced the rate of lung cancer, the reality was that, despite them stopping smoking, their rates had still increased.

Burch's findings also link in with the smoking /illness/social class issue. His data showed that between 1955 and 1971 the risk of lung cancer amongst all men in England and Wales more than doubled (an increase of over 100%) whilst the risk amongst doctors increased by only 31%. Doctors are part of the higher social classes and as such tend to be healthier. In the same paper, Burch also plotted cigarette consumption for both men and women in England and Wales against lung cancer death rates (LCDRs) between 1890 and 1971. His data showed that the largest increases in LCDRs in both sexes were between 1916-1920 and 1931-1935, yet during these times the number of female smokers in England and Wales was very small. This led Burch to conclude that the rise in lung cancer was actually due to improved diagnosis rather than smoking. In other words, there were not more cases of lung cancer as such, there were just more cases being recognised.

Furthermore, in England and Wales there was a thirty year gap between the time men started smoking and the time women started smoking. This is why the oft-spoken anti-smoking mantra, that there is a thirty year incubation period of smoking causing lung cancer, surfaced. They claim this is why the rates of female lung cancers increased decades after they began smoking, rather than synonymously. However, Burch's work refutes this, too, as he plotted lung cancer rates for males in 1906-1926, and female rates for 1936-1966 and showed that the two graph lines were entirely dissimilar – whereas they would be synchronous if the incubation theory was true.

Chapter three mentioned that Doll and Hill conducted a study which highlighted an inverse correlation of lung cancer between inhalers and non-inhalers. The study was in fact the aforementioned London Hospital's study and it classified smokers as inhaling vs. non-inhaling. Page 188 of the 1964 Surgeon General's report references a "negative association" between inhaling and lung cancer, based on the Doll/Hill study. In 1959, Ronald Fisher, the father of modern statistics, analysed some of the data from the study and concluded that there was a lower rate of lung cancer in inhalers than non-inhalers.[81] This highlights the obvious point, and what could be crucial to the whole debate about smoking and cancer: breathing smoke into the lungs does not cause lung cancer. This leads to the question 'if inhaling smoke does not cause lung cancer, how does smoking cause it?' Perhaps this alone shows that smoking does not cause lung cancer. For anyone wondering, the way Doll got around this discrepancy in the Doctor's study was to simply stop asking participants if they inhaled or not. Fisher had this to say:

> Should not these workers have let the world know not only that they had discovered the cause of lung cancer (cigarettes) but also that they had discovered the means of its prevention (inhaling cigarette smoke)? How had the MRC [Medical Research Council] the heart to withhold this information from the thousands who would otherwise die of lung cancer?

This remark was offered facetiously to point out the errors Doll had encountered; the finding that smoking 'caused' lung cancer was as statistically significant as the result that inhaling 'prevented' lung cancer. It reaffirms the lack of objectivity when one takes into account that Doll chose to not take this finding into account, despite its statistical significance. Had the work been truly objective then he would have commenced further research into that area, or at least acknowledged the possibility it was correct. Instead, though, he simply omitted the inhalation question from further questionnaires.

Doll conducted a follow-up to his Doctor's study, released in 2004.[82] The study tells us that most of the doctors who only smoked cigarettes at the time of the original study had stopped by the time of the follow-up study – actually, we are told only 6% had continued to smoke. Despite us knowing this, Doll still tried to estimate the number of pack years smoked by those who stopped smoking in an attempt to develop correlations to lung cancer. Of course, Doll could only do this by the recollections of those

---

[81] Fischer R.A; (1959) *Smoking, The Cancer Controversy, Some Attempts to Assess the Evidence*, Edinburg; Oliver and Boyd

[82] http://www.bmj.com/cgi/content/full/309/6959/901

interviewed by mail at infrequent follow-ups as to how long they had smoked and when they gave up. The problem this poses is recall bias – a problem that prospective studies are designed to avoid. The approach also requires the researcher to make numerous adjustments to take into account the effects of smoking cessation – adjustments which allowed Doll's biases to get in the way of objective analysis. Even more damaging is the quote mentioned already in this chapter, where Doll said in 2001 at the termination of this study that it was: "devised by Sir Austin Bradford Hill to achieve maximum publicity for the critical link between smoking and lung cancer".

Sir Richard Doll was involved in other studies, none of which do him any favours. Unfortunately, Doll's findings on smoking and cancer gave him enormous rewards and success to the tune of a knighthood, an Oxford University building researching cancer named after him during his lifetime, freedom of the city of Oxford, international awards, and the fact that he dominated the British cancer epidemiology scene for over 50 years. However, what is now clear is that at least some portion, and perhaps much, of his work in this area has been strongly criticised as fraudulent and, besides the work on smoking, his lack of integrity that allowed him to work for the companies that he did may well be responsible for the lack of knowledge and, in turn, lack of warnings, on certain products that could have saved millions of lives worldwide.

Despite this information now being known, and the article published in the *Guardian* as previously mentioned, this reality is entirely ignored by the medical establishment and government. Perhaps one day it will get the attention it deserves and people will reassess his smoking/cancer studies and realise that, actually, they do not prove smoking causes cancer, they are nothing more than purpose-made results from a hypothesis that did not set out to discover the effects of smoking, but to prove smoking as harmful – two entirely different things. If I wanted to prove that something caused cancer, I could easily do it by simply selecting a product, and then manipulating the controls and factors within the study to produce the desired results.

There are two particular scientific publications which need a mention, *The Causes of Cancer: Quantitative Estimates of Avoidable*

*Risks of Cancer in the United States Today* (1981)[83] which Doll wrote with Professor Richard Peto, and *Effects of exposure to vinyl chloride. An Assessment of the Evidence* (1988)[84] which he wrote alone. These have been regarded for a long time by leading scientists as using evidence which might be deemed to massively underplay the risks by using parameters which are obviously wrong.

For instance, the 1981 study written with Peto was supposed to cover all environmental and work-related cancers, yet African-Americans and anyone aged over sixty were deliberately omitted from the statistics. This is despite the fact that exposure would be expected to be higher among blue collar workers and the poor where African-Americans might be deemed to be over-represented because of the locations they lived and worked in. As for old people, the cancer incidence would without a doubt be expected to be highest in the old. To summarise: Doll had a specific result in mind and he knew what factors would alter those results, so he left them out. Unbiased, fair and professional research? Not in the least.

The same tactic was employed in the 1988 study which he wrote on his own, regarding vinyl chloride. In this study, older workers, who had heavy exposure to the chemical given their many years working with it, and plants regarded as particularly dangerous were all excluded, whilst young workers, who had little to no exposure, were included, thus producing results that showed there was little to no risk of the product in question.

As mentioned before, Doll was receiving vast payments from Monsanto and other companies for his work, but there is more. Doll's personal archive reveals that Doll himself, and the Oxford college he founded – Green College – were receiving very large sums of money from Turner and Newall, the asbestos company, and the industry body the Chemical Manufacturers Association, on top of the aforementioned Monsanto payments. Just how vast were these sums of money? Turner and Newall were giving payments of £50,000 to Green College; there was a thirty year financial relationship between Turner and Newall and Sir

---

[83] Doll et. al, (1981)*The Causes of Cancer: Quantitative Estimates of Avoidable Risks of Cancer in the United States Today* Journal of the National Cancer Institute 66

[84] Doll (1988) *Effects of exposure to vinyl chloride. An assessment of the evidence" Scand J Work Environ Health*

Richard Doll; and payments of between £12,000 and 15,000 to Doll from the Chemical Manufacturers' Association.

Incredibly, the story does not end there. In 1982, there was an exposé on the dangers of asbestos and Doll was there at factory meetings, on request of Turner and Newall, with workers across Britain to reassure them that their danger risk from exposure to asbestos was minimal. Doll's, and Turner and Newall's, own figures at the time put the cancer risk incidence at one in forty which is notably high, but, not surprisingly, the incidence now has been shown to be much higher – in Britain, there are between 1900 and 2000 annual deaths from mesothlioma, a cancer apparently caused solely by exposure to asbestos fibre.[85] That figure is also doubled by other lung cancer deaths caused by asbestos.

Going back to the 1981 study conducted by Doll and Peto, the Health and Safety Executive still quotes the results of that study as the basis for their:

> current best estimate of the proportion of cancer deaths in Great Britain due to occupational exposures over the last few decades as 4%, with an associated uncertainty range of 5% to 8%.[86]

It is only now that there is work underway to update it. Their study was considered groundbreaking at the time because it proved that environmental and occupational causes of cancer represented only 4% of total cancer mortality, when even consultants to what was the Chemical Manufacturer's Association (the company paying Doll) had admitted the incidence was probably 20%.

As for the 1988 article on vinyl chloride, Doll reported that there was no significant risk associated with the product other than in the liver. However, the report failed to mention the payments Doll was receiving from the chemical companies. According to the ACC in 2001, speaking of the paper,

---

[85] http://www.prlog.org/10071014-mesothlioma-com-announces-site-launch.html

[86] http://www.hse.gov.uk/statistics/causdis/cancer.htm

the world's leading researchers have studied vinyl chloride and brain cancer and concluded that the evidence does not support a link between brain cancer and vinyl chloride.

Something else that they did not mention was that the article had been reviewed by Ted Torkelson, medical advisor to Dow and Geoffrey Paddle, another chemical industry funded medic.

Swedish cancer expert Dr Lennart Hardell said:

> At the time many scientists were suspicious that the reports seemed to be too pro-industry. Many wondered if he had close links with industry and were concerned with some of his findings because his conclusions formed the basis for health and safety guidelines and legislation many people have died unnecessarily in my opinion.[87]

The unnecessary victims of vinyl chloride Hardell was talking about include the workers of Vinatex PVC in Derbyshire. It was a joint venture between American company Conoco and a British company called Staveley Chemicals Ltd. Vinatex PVC opened in 1969 and converted Vinyl Chloride Monomer to PVC, and when it went out of business in 1984 dozens of Vinatex workers exposed to vinyl chloride were either dead or dying. Doll may have decided that there was no significant risk associated with vinyl chloride but research by Trade Unions in Derbyshire estimate that about 40% of the 280 workers at the factory are now dead, and many of these deaths were from rare forms of cancer. Sir Richard Doll was closely connected with both the Imperial Cancer Research Fund and Cancer Research and the two, now merged, have located their Cancer Research UK Epidemiology Unit (CEU) alongside part of the Department of Public Health and the University's Clinical Trial Service Unit & Epidemiological Studies Unit (CTSU) in the Richard Doll Building.[88]

The 4% figure that Doll and Peto reached translates to 6,000 deaths attributable to occupational/environmental cancer in the UK – to put this into context, it is twice the number of annual deaths from roads and twenty times those killed in workplace

---

[87] http://www.injurywatch.co.uk/

[88] Ibid.

accidents. Despite this being a high number in itself, other researchers in the area thought the figure seemed low and Doll and Peto themselves admitted their researches were guesses, saying that it was "impossible to make any precise attempt at the proportion of cancers that are attributable to hazards at work".[89]

There are also many other problems with their research: there were a number of cancers that were missing entirely from their analysis or were claimed to be not work-related, including melanoma and breast cancer (which is the most common cancer amongst women); overall risks to women would be under-estimated because of their relatively late entry to the industrial workforce in large numbers; prostate cancer, the most prevalent cancer amongst men, was only considered a risk for cadmium-exposed workers, despite studies that have linked prostate cancer to exposure to pesticides, metalworking fluids and other occupational exposures. The study only included sixteen substances or industries thought to be carcinogenic to humans, which is a fraction of the true number – the International Agency on Research on Cancer classifies eighty-nine substances as definite human carcinogens, sixty-four as probable carcinogens and 264 as possible human carcinogens. The report only considered mortality and not morbidity (number of cases), which is a considerably higher figure – even the 4% figure, which translates to 6,000 deaths, would in actuality mean 11,000 cases a year. Cancers in those over sixty-five years old were excluded, which dramatically reduced the number of cancers considered (recent figures showing that cancer deaths under sixty amounted to only 26% of the total), and this alone may have reduced the work cancer toll to less than half the real number. Cancers in those working in small industries were excluded; the analysis missed out those with indirect exposures to carcinogens, for example maintenance workers in contact with asbestos, which are now amongst the highest risk for asbestos cancer in the UK. Moreover, the study only considered human evidence – but for some substances and industries the studies had not been conducted, but there was strong evidence from the toxicological and animal studies – as a result many cancers caused or related to workplace exposures would have switched columns to lifestyle, smoking or other causation categories. Finally, non-Hodgkin's lymphoma, which is considered to be one of the most common work-related cancers,

---

[89] Ibid.

was classified as having only a slight risk association impacting on relatively few workers.[90]  Dr James Brophy, Executive Director of OHCOW, a Canadian occupational cancer clinic, said of the study:

> Companies were ecstatic because it posed the whole cancer thing politically as a matter of lifestyle. That had consequences for prevention in that it effectively ended any chance of a structured and well resourced strategy to combat cancer worldwide.

Another major review of the environmental and occupational causes of cancer produced in 2005 concluded:

> It is difficult to estimate the difficulty of Doll and Peto's views but their 1981 article had been cited in over 440 other scientific articles by 2004. More importantly, it has been cited repeatedly by commentators who argue that 'cleaning up the environment' is not going to make much difference in cancer rates.[91]

The study, co-authored by Dr Richard Clapp of the University of Boston Medical School, estimates that the occupational cancer incidence figure given by Doll/Peto probably underestimates the real figure by a factor of between two and four, suggesting the real figure for occupational cancer is between 8% and 16%. This would mean anything up to 43,200 cancer cases annually.[92]  The only positive to come out of these studies is that we can see, again, that those in the lower classes are more at risk. Factory workers will tend to be from a lower economic status and as such be at risk with the chemicals, as well as the stress of the job, long hours, and low wages which mean poorer quality food and reduced healthcare treatment.

---

[90] Epstein, S.S; (2003) *Stop Cancer Before It Starts: How to Win the War On Cancer* Environmental and Occupational Medicine UIC

[91] Richard Clapp *et al* (2005) *Environmental and Occupational Causes of Cancer: A Review of Recent Scientific Literature* Lowell Center for Sustainable Production, University of Massachusetts Lowell, September

[92] www.injurywatch.co.uk

Before leaving this chapter, I will give some more information on Doll's less than impressive history: in 1983 he claimed that lead in petroleum vehicle exhaust had no correlation with increased lead levels and learning disabilities in children, a result that undoubtedly had some roots in the fact that General Motors had funded the study. In 1987, in light of childhood leukaemia clusters near fifteen nuclear power plants and evidence showing a 21% excess of lymphoid leukaemia in children and young adults living within ten miles of the power plants, Doll dismissed the evidence and claimed that "over clean" homes of nuclear workers rendered their children susceptible to unidentified leukaemia viruses. In 1988 Doll claimed that the mortality from leukaemia and multiple myeloma among servicemen exposed to radiation from atom bomb tests was a "statistical quirk", and in 1993 he revisited the study to eliminate the majority of cases which developed within two years of exposure, claiming that such short latency disproved any possible causal relation. In 1991 he said:

> Young people say smoking cannot be all that bad or the Government would never allow it to be promoted in the way it does...I accept that millions of pounds are at stake, but no price can be put on the misery and suffering of smokers who die of cancer and of their families and friends who are forced to watch one of the most painful ways of dying.

This is a shocking statement from a man who spent his career manipulating evidence to protect his own interests and possibly subject countless people to the misery of disease and suffering. There is plenty more that can be exposed about the late, great pioneer of cancer Sir Richard Doll, but enough has been shown to highlight the fact that a significant portion of his work should be regarded as invalid. The British Doctor's study itself was flawed from the outset by using statistical data based on respondent participants, and thanks to Burch it has now been entirely disproved, while the London Hospital's study had numerous problems which completely invalidated Doll's results and conclusion. In short, while Doll may well remain the leading figure in the anti-smoking crusade his breakthrough study is nothing more than misleading and wrong: while his own results claimed a reduction of cancer in former smokers the true figure was a 31% increase. Finally, to shed some light on his findings, Doll claimed that smokers had a twenty-four times greater risk of contracting lung cancer than non-smokers, with 160 in 100,000 smokers getting cancer compared to seven in 100,000 non-smokers. However, whilst this is presented in a scary way, it actually means that the chance of a smoker *not* getting lung cancer is still 99.8%.

Surgeon General's Report 1964

As mentioned in chapter two, the 1964 Surgeon General's Report was issued by ten scientists who used a selection of prospective studies to issue their report. A handful of the studies were as follows:[93]

(1) British doctors, a questionnaire having been sent to all members of the medical profession in the UK. *Doll and Hill.* (1956)
(2) White American men in nine states, enrolled by American Cancer Association volunteers, each of whom enlisted ten white males between fifty and sixty years of age. *Hammond and Horn.* (1958)
(3) Policy holders of US Government Life Insurance policies. *Dorn.* (1958)
(4) Men, 35-64, in nine occupations in California which were suspected of having a high occupational risk of lung cancer. *Dunn, Linden and Breslow.* (1960)
(5) California members of the American Legion and their wives. *Dunn, Buell, and Breslow.* (1961)
(6) Canadian War Veterans. *Best, Josie and Walker.* (1961)
(7) American men in ten states, enrolled by volunteers from the American Cancer society, each of whom was asked to enroll about ten families containing at least one person over forty-five. *Hammond.* (1963)

As with Doll's study (which appears at the top of this list), there was an immediate problem: the response rate. Taking the five studies for which it had data on the non-response rate, the Committee concluded that the average non-response rate was about 32%. This is approximately a third, and a number large enough to dramatically alter the results. As such the results must be viewed with caution. After all, if a study is conducted with only twenty people, it cannot be generalised and people will be reluctant to

---

[93] 1964 Surgeon General's Report

accept the findings, however a study with 200 participants has a lot more validity. The more participants a study has, the more valid the results, and when a third of the possible response population is not partaking there can be a dramatic difference in the results. On page 116 of the Report the Committee cited a paper by Berkson:[94]

> The death rate in the complete population (3,000) was 42% higher than the respondent death rate. The non-smoker death rate was over 38 times as high among non-respondents as among respondents (60.1221/1.553), whereas among smokers it was only 1.8 times as high. [Berkson's] calculations referred to an early year of the study, in which the differential entry of ill persons among smokers and non-smokers are likely to be most marked. Further, as we interpret his writing, the example was intended as a warning against the type of subtle bias that can arise whenever a study has a high proportion of non respondents, rather than a claim that this numerical estimate of the bias actually applied to these studies.

What this shows is exactly what has been mentioned: skewed results. Berkson is saying that the death rate amongst non-responding non-smokers was thirty-eight times as great as the rate amongst responding non-smokers, and the death rate among non-responding smokers was only 1.8 times as great as the death rate among corresponding respondents. It is very obvious to anyone who cares to read that information that such a discrepancy will almost certainly lead to one-sided results. Amazingly (or perhaps not so amazingly in light of their desire to support their hypothesis), the Committee decided to claim the finding bore no relevance and even implied, without saying it directly, that they did not think Berkson meant what he wrote.. This serves to show, again, that there is much bias present and that these studies are flawed. It is also clear that the researchers had a clear agenda. As mentioned in chapter two, the members of the Committee leave a lot to be desired and it is a curious point that there was no statistician present.

---

[94] Berkson, J. *The Statistical Study of Association Between Smoking and Lung Cancer*. Proc. Staff Meeting, Mayo Clin

As has been shown more than once, socio-economic status appears to have a strong link to the onset of disease. The Committee also picked up on this: table twenty-six on page 109 of the report shows incidents of morbidity derived from all seven prospective studies for twenty-five different causes of death. With the exception of cancer of the rectum and intestines, smokers showed a statistically increased risk of death compared to non-smokers. It was also claimed that smokers are more likely to die from accidents and suicide, as well as cirrhosis of the liver and bladder cancer, than non-smokers. This goes to show that statistics prove nothing, as no one would say that smokers are generally significantly more likely to die from accidents simply because they smoked. Therefore, a statistical link between smoking and lung cancer is not necessarily indicative of a causative effect.

Indeed, Brownlee was troubled by these findings as he failed to see the "specificity" of smoking to the disease which the Committee claimed to be "caused" by smoking i.e. lung cancer. One thing that is often missing in the field of smoking is logic, and logic would suggest there is no connection between smoking and prostate cancer or liver cirrhosis. Thus, these findings really show a link between social class and disease and death. As previously mentioned, those from the lower classes have more menial and dangerous jobs, and as such are more likely to be involved in accidents – either at work or on the road if that is what the job entails. They are also more likely to suffer from depression. Cigarette smokers tend to come from the lower classes, whilst cigar and pipe smokers tend to come from the higher classes, and statistically cigar and pipe smokers outlive non-smokers. Perhaps, then, the statistic that cigarette smokers are more likely to contract lung cancer is really because they tend to be from the lower social classes, rather than because they choose to smoke. Somewhat surprisingly, Doll himself acknowledged that diet has a bearing on cancer, claiming that the carcinogenic effects of smoking could be affected by diet: smokers who consumed above average levels of beta carotene – a vitamin present in carrots – could lower their risk of lung cancer by an estimated 40%. This adds weight to the social class argument, as those from the higher classes are more likely to consume high quality food than those from the lower classes.

So, then, the committee did indeed acknowledge the possibility of bias due to social class. However, it appears they entirely ignored the possibility of detection bias.

With regards to the studies themselves, all the living participants involved knew what was being studied (smoking and disease), and so did their doctors. They all knew that the researchers were hypothesising that smoking causes cancer. Consequently, because of the faith people place in scientists, everybody involved was simply waiting for the smokers to develop lung cancer. This would have increased the chances of detection bias, yet this was not mentioned in the Committee's conclusion. It is also worth noting that the methodology the studies followed was calculated to exaggerate the possibility of detection bias because the researchers were out to prove smoking causes cancer. As mentioned before, there is a big difference between setting out to prove something and setting out to discover the effects objectively. This is the entire basis upon which the need for double-blind scientific experimentation is founded.

Regarding the point that the methodology was calculated to exaggerate the possibility of detection bias, Doll's study of British Doctor's is a good example. All deaths in which lung cancer was a contributing cause were classified as deaths *from* lung cancer, even though the direct cause of death may have been something else (page 101 of the Report). It is interesting, then, that this study was the one which purported to show smoking was the highest risk for lung cancer.[95]

One of the seven aforementioned studies is referred to in the Report as "Men in Twenty-five States" study, also known as the Million Person Study or the Hammond and Horn study. The Introduction mentioned the bias present in studies and how anti-smoking studies are funded by those with interests in specific results. This is no exception and it was conducted by the American Cancer Society. Between October 1959 and February 1960, the ACS enrolled men in a smoker survey. The survey worked by asking female volunteers to pick ten family members among their acquaintances, each with at least one person over the age of forty-five, and note if they died during the survey period of

---

[95] Vandenbroucke J.P. (1991) *Invited Commentary: How Much Retropsychology?* Vol 133, Number 5 *American Journal of Epidemiology* "The original case-control studies by Wynder and Graham and by Doll and Hill are still used in a famous epidemiologic exercise....where they serve as examples of what can go wrong: biased ascertainment of exposure, selection of cases and controls from different source populations, poor ascertainment of caseness, etc..."

approximately twenty-two months. More specifically they were told to find out if the cause of death was lung cancer.

The study had 448,000 useable replies, representing the same number of men between thirty-five and eighty-nine years of age. Whilst we know the number of useable replies, we do not know how many replies were rejected as unusable because each volunteer was free to use her own criteria. Another piece of information we are left without is how many smokers were studied as opposed to non-smokers because the results do not contain such information. As mentioned earlier, missing data means that results could have been drastically different and can bring the validity of the study into question. Accordingly, the lung cancer rates are quite meaningless for the study if it is not known who smoked and who did not. What we do know is that during the time period of twenty-two months there was a total of 11,612, which is a figure much lower than the overall death rate for white males. The Surgeon General acknowledged this and claimed that the participants in the survey were considerably healthier than the average person. It is highly unlikely that the study consisted of almost half a million of the healthiest people in the country, especially considering the age of the men ranged from thirty-five to eighty-nine, as a large percentage of the survey population were elderly and at a higher risk for death and cancer. It is not a valid measure to include those in their eighties with those in their thirtiess, because the elderly are much more likely to contract disease or die than their younger counterparts. The increased rates of the elderly are lumped in with the rates of the younger participants and provide a misleading result. Instead, there is a different conclusion lurking within the study data. It observed the mortality ratios for different types of smokers, as opposed to non-smokers, which were:

Cigarettes only 1.83; Cigarettes and other 1.54; Cigars only 0.97; Pipes only 0.86

This, again, adds to the large body of evidence showing that social class plays a large role, as cigar and pipe smokers outlived non-smokers despite exposure to larger amounts of tobacco smoke and the chemicals within it. This is the same result as found in Doll's study. Statistically, this could be used to show cigar and pipe smoking are protective against cancer and, to an extreme based on the data, death. This is unlikely to be the case so something else must be the real reason for the data, and I feel that is social class. Cigar and pipe smokers tend to be from the upper classes, and cigarette smokers from the lower classes. Suppose for a moment smoking, in any form, is a harmless factor that has no bearing on mortality, and we may get nearer the truth. In actuality, it appears that this is the case and smoking studies do little else than to add weight to the theory that it is lifestyle and diet of people that affects the onset of diseases such as cancer, which is reflected in the mortality rates of the smokers as we can get an idea of the social classes they come from.

The Report does not list the number of lung cancer deaths which were recorded by the volunteers in the study, instead the results of this study were put together with the other six looked at here, including Doll's Doctor's study. Most or all of these studies were organised by the cancer societies, with Doll's being a noticeable exception. The results of all seven studies show there were 26,223 smoker deaths and 11,168 non-smoker deaths. Of these, there were 1,833 cancer deaths in smokers and only 123 in non-smokers, producing a mortality ratio of 10.8 for death from lung cancer among smokers as opposed to non-smokers. Table fifteen of the Report shows that for all the various studies, the age-adjusted death rates for the study subjects were much lower than the age adjusted death rate of 22.9 per 1000 man years for US white males in 1960. In the Twenty-five States study, the death rate for non-smokers was 12.8, compared to 18.5 for smokers of less than a pack a day and 19.2 for those who smoked over a pack a day. These results are very similar to the other five studies (Doll's being omitted), however the Twenty-five States one had a footnote which said "these results may be too low by about 1.7% since the person-years used in the computation included some contribution by men who had not been fully traced".

Table two of the Report gives the mortality ratios for current smokers for various studies including the Twenty-five States study. The Surgeon General also tells us that the figures were age adjusted, which leads us to believe that all figures given in the Report are age adjusted and represent current smokers. However, this is not the case.

Table nineteen shows the number of deaths from each of twenty-five different causes ranging from lung cancer to cancer of the intestines. The figures given in this table represent the sums of all of the deaths recorded in all of the seven studies and there is a footnote saying "current cigarettes only for four studies: all cigarettes (current and ex-) for the two California studies and Men in Twenty-five States". This may appear to be straightforward and worthwhile, however "ex-" means that not only current smokers are classed as smokers, but anyone who has ever smoked. This bears a huge significance as it is not objective analysis. This has spectacular bearing as in 1961, around the same time the studies were conducted and exactly the same time the Twenty-five States study was carried out, over half of American men smoked. This means that over half were continuing smokers and, as we all know, many people try smoking, are social smokers, or smoke and stop at a later date. This means that, using the Report's method of including anyone who has ever smoked as a smoker, the statistic of the smoking population would be incredibly high. Thus, it is no surprise that 90% of the lung cancer deaths occurred in smokers. Furthermore, with such a large number of people smoking it is a certainty that there will be a large percentage of various diseases present in smokers. This is not because of the smoking, but because there are more smokers than non-smokers. With smokers making up the majority of the population it is quite obvious they are going to have statistically higher incidents of disease and mortality. It is much the same as saying Caucasians in England statistically suffer more disease than non-Caucasians people; this is a very obvious point because Caucasians make up the vast majority of the English population.

One huge problem with the Report was merging the results of all seven studies together to produce a singular result. Each study had different methodologies and as such the results were relevant only to the particular study. Each study had different age groups and populations (including social classes, jobs, gender etc.), all of which make it difficult, if not impossible, to lump all the results together. Unfortunately, the only way we could truly see what each study found and assess it individually would be to have the results of each study. That information is not available and, given that the Report is over forty years old, it probably never will be.

It is worth noting that the Surgeon General was alarmed by the fact that there were so few deaths during the study period compared to the deaths that would occur in a cross section of white males on a national level. The footnote saying the figures from the "Men in Twnety-five States" study were low is essentially pointless as all six studies from the cancer studies yielded results that were in the same region. However, the Committee still spent a considerable passage of time discussing the discrepancy, suggesting that, besides other reasons, the people who were already sick might not have been chosen as study participants by the female volunteers. This is a very valid point and was probably part of the reason. Sadly, though, it does not affect the overall conclusion of the Report, and rather than compile a second Report or redo a particular study the Committee published it regardless.

There is also another possible reason for the low death rate that the Committee failed to mention. The Surgeon General wrote in the Report that the females who conducted the study by finding the volunteers were free to weed out any responses which they felt to be inappropriate. The Surgeon General also reported that the women were expected to obtain a death certificate for each death they reported. A possible explanation for the low death rate is the women simply did not report all the deaths so they could avoid getting a death certificate, as they are a lot of trouble to obtain. The women may have decided it was not worth reporting all of them or, more likely, given the study was on smoking the women may have felt that if the deceased died as a result of something unrelated to smoking the death was simply not relevant and thus not worth reporting.

Whatever the reason, the fact remains that the death rate for the study was, as the Committee admitted, low enough to raise alarm bells, meaning that the Report should not have been considered conclusive enough to make any real assumptions or decisions.

<u>2004 Surgeon General's Report</u>

There are many Surgeon General's Reports looking at smoking, and each one is just as flawed as the last one. In fact, nearly each one tells of new diseases that smoking causes and the 2004 Report has the Surgeon General concluding "smoking harms nearly every organ of the body, causing many diseases and reducing the health of smokers in general" and citing new studies which leave him in no doubt that there are now more diseases to add to the ever-growing list of smoking-related risks. These include cancer of the pancreas, larynx, bladder, stomach, cervix, kidney and oral cavity, as well as abdominal aortic aneurysm, acute myeloid leukaemia, cataracts, pneumonia and periodontitis.

It seems that the word 'cause' either has lost all meaning, or people simply do not know how to use it. If I light a match and put it to paper, I will with all certainty 'cause' a fire. For something to be a causative agent, it means that, with all certainty, that product will lead to that result e.g. lit match to paper causes fire. If, as anti-smokers postulate, smoking *causes* cancer of various organs, then the rates of said cancers would all be very similar, as they are 'caused' by smoking. Furthermore, the statistical rates of disease caused by smoking would be very similar in every nation with smoking. However, this is not the case at all. What these extra diseases also mean is that, with tobacco causing so many diseases and deaths the world over, there would be an absolute epidemic of a variety of cancers, and during the post-war period where over half of the American male population smoked there really would have been serious population depletion. Given the aerodigestive tract (the combined organs and tissues of the respiratory tract and the upper part of the digestive tract, including the lips, mouth, tongue, nose, throat, vocal cords, and part of the oesophagus and windpipe) is exposed to higher concentrations of smoke than the lungs, one would expect there to be higher incidence of cancers of the mouth, tongue, and oesophagus. Apparently this is not the case, leading to the realisation that the anti-smoking crusade should have put some forethought into their plan when they first linked smoking to lung cancer. It is also a point that Doll and subsequent researchers should have thought of when they became convinced by their flawed data.

On page 324 of the Report, the Surgeon General says that "smoking causes genetic changes in cells of the lung that ultimately lead to the development of lung cancer". This is unlikely to be true, given the fact that pathologists admit they cannot tell the difference between a smoker's lung and a non-smoker's lung, and that no animal study has ever succeeded in inducing lung cancer with tobacco smoke. We must also not forget that if smoking caused a genetic change then researchers would undoubtedly be able to recognise smoking-induced lung cancer as a different type of lung cancer – but they cannot. On the same page, the Surgeon General shoots himself in the foot once again: "lung cancer incidence and mortality rates in men are now declining, reflecting past patterns of cigarette use, while rates in women are still rising". First and foremost, smoking rates dropped significantly from the 1960s onwards yet lung cancer rates increased even more significantly. If lung cancer rates really have started to decline it certainly is not a result of smoking cessation, as this would have appeared decades ago; even if we accept the incubation theory, rates would have fallen sharply around the 1990s. Secondly, it is very likely, if not a certainty, that with the falling rates of smoking, detection bias will rear its head again as people, including doctors, *expect* there to be less incidence of lung cancer with less smoking, and thus they will not be looking for it.

One last point, referring to that previous quote, on page sixty-two of the Report the Surgeon General also says that, speaking of cancers of the oral cavity and pharynx, "incidence rates are more than twice as high in men as in women". These two quotes completely contradict each other: apparently, men smoking less has resulted in them suffering less lung cancer whilst women, in their refusal to give up, are still suffering from lung cancer. At the same time, though, men are suffering from twice as much oral cancer than women – as a result of smoking! It seems as though no one was around to proof-read the Report before it was released, because if they had surely such remarks would have been discovered and omitted.

The problem with the studies that convince the Surgeon General is that they are all retrospective, which means the victim, or relative of the deceased, are questioned regarding the victim's/ deceased's smoking habits. One need not be a scientist to realise that retrospective studies are inherently flawed and lead to recall bias. This is where the interviewee is likely to exaggerate their smoking habits with the notion that they must have smoked heavily or they would not have contracted the illness which led to their demise. Another problem is, of course, that remembering how many cigarettes someone smoked thirty years ago is not an easy task and there is no way the response can be accurate. In fact, in the 1964 Surgeon General's Report the authors rejected the retrospective studies and focused on the remaining studies; it speaks volumes that forty years on the medical establishment now accepts flawed methodologies that were rejected in the past for being unreliable.

Another major problem with the Report is that most of the studies were adjusted in ways that are unnecessary. Age adjustments happen all the time and this is for the valid reason that disease rates amongst the elderly are not comparable with disease rates of young adults. However, other things adjusted for included educational attainment, alcohol consumption, geographic residence and, of all things, religion. Now, *examining* those things is one thing, and worthwhile – education and geographic residence, in particular, could point towards social status or pollution exposure, but studying something is not the same as adjusting for it. In fact, it is not at all clear *how* such adjustments were made i.e. on what grounds and by how much and whether at least some of those adjustments may have been made on the basis of either unconscious expectations/biases of the researchers or even a conscious effort to bring the results into line with what the researchers felt they 'knew' to be the 'truth.'

One study of particular noteworthiness is a Brazilian hospital based study looking at cancer of the aerodigestive tract. What makes it so interesting is that it adjusted for "cumulative alcohol and tobacco use, race, beverage temperature, religion, wood stove use, and consumption of spicy foods". It is not a stupid question to ask 'why would spicy foods consumption or wood stove use be factors?' and the wood stove use seems suspiciously as though a non-smoker with cancer of the aerodigestive tract who used a wood stove would be omitted from the study on the basis that the wood smoke was responsible for the onset of the disease. More important, though, is the fact that the patients had been computer matched beforehand with controls for gender, age and their admission times, so no further adjustments were needed. The fact that such adjustments were made brings in to question the objectivity of the researchers.

Finally, the studies produce conflicting results from each other. For example some concluded that smokers of low tar cigarettes had less chance of contracting lung cancer than smokers of higher yielding brands, whilst others concluded that:

> After adjusting for age and total pack years, the difference in risk was insignificant [because] low-tar smokers compensated by smoking almost half a pack more per day.

Given the discrepancies amongst the studies, there is little room for doubt that the Surgeon General's conclusion that smoking caused a range of new diseases was simply propaganda adhering to the politically correct view that smoking is harmful; after all, he had no basis to make a 'conclusive' statement as the studies themselves did not produce a unified conclusion.

Ernst Wynder M.D.

Wynder was mentioned in chapter two regarding his use of lung photographs, which he used to try and prove that the lung of a smoker is black as a result of tobacco tar. Wynder had been crusading against smoking since the 1950s and in February 1991 his paper *Comparative Epidemiology of Cancer Between the United States and Japan*[96] was published in the journal *Cancer*. The study set out with the assumption that smoking causes lung cancer – much the same as the study funded by the ACS mentioned in the Introduction – and was funded by the National Cancer Institute and the American Cancer Society Special Institutional.

The study contains a graph, showing cigarette consumption per capita of the USA and Japan between 1920 and 1985. The graph relies upon data plotted at five year intervals and attempts to show a sharp decrease in cigarette consumption during the Second World War (1939-1945) to less than a third of the consumption before the war. The graph also, somehow, tries to show that for the whole period of 1920 to 1985 the Japanese had a lower consumption than the USA. I must now borrow an excerpt from Lauren Colby, author of *In Defense of Smokers*,[97] as he points out a basic problem in epidemiology of the difficulty of comparing data for two differing populations:

> Suppose we postulate that people who eat jellybeans are prone to develop more carbuncles than people who don't. To test the theory, we decide to study jellybean consumption in two different countries: country A and country B. Both countries have populations of 1,000,000 divided equally between men and women. Jellybean consumption in both countries is 1,000,000 beans per day, yielding a per capita consumption figure of one jellybean per person per day.
>
> There is, however, a difference. In Country A, only men eat jellybeans, while in Country B, both men and women eat jellybeans. Obviously, in Country A, the jellybean consumption for men is 2 per day, while in Country B it is one. In Country A, the daily jellybean

---

[96] http://www.ncbi.nlm.nih.gov/pubmed/1985768

[97] Colby, L; (1999) *In Defense of Smokers* http://www.lcolby.com/b-chap5.htm

consumption for women is zero, while in country B it is one. Any comparison of the two countries must take this into account.

The researchers, Wynder et al, presented data on relative smoking rates for both genders of Japan and the United States, and the rates are expressed in terms of the percentage of each sex who smoke:

| Year: | 1955 | 1965 | 1976 | 1980 | 1985 |
|---|---|---|---|---|---|
| U . S . Males | 52.6 | 52.1 | 41.6 | 37.9 | 33.2 |
| U . S . Females | 24.5 | 34.2 | 32.5 | 29.8 | 27.9 |
| Japanese Males | 81.4 | 82.3 | 75.1 | 70.2 | 64.6 |
| Japanese Females | 12.8 | 17.7 | 15.4 | 14.4 | 13.7 |

Despite the researchers claim that the Japanese consumed less cigarettes than Americans, their own data clearly shows the Japanese smoked far more.

The researchers also presented statistics for 1970, 1980, and 1986, showing that Japanese males smoke more cigarettes than American males whilst Japanese females smoke fewer than American women. The total consumption figures given in the report's graph need to be adjusted to account for the differing rates of smoking between men and women in both countries, however this adjustment was not made. If it had been made, the graph would have shown a far higher consumption in Japan than in the USA because in the official graph the low rates of smoking Japanese women brings down the total of female smokers, yet if the adjustment had been made this would no longer be so.

The report also included data comparing lung cancer death rates (LCDRs) in Japan and the USA, although only figures for Caucasian American males and females were included, omitting African-Americans and American-Indians. No reason is stated for this, but it is most likely due to the fact that these groups of people suffer less lung cancer than their Caucasian counterparts and would have skewed the results the researchers were trying to obtain. The male LCDRs, age adjusted, per 100,000 of the population were:

| Year | 1955 | 1965 | 1975 | 1985 |
|------|------|------|------|------|
| U.S. | 90 | 130 | 160 | 165 |
| Japan | 15 | 35 | 45 | 50 |

What is apparent from this table and the previous table is that whilst rates of cigarette consumption (for males of both Japan and the USA) decreased steadily over the relevant years, the lung cancer rates increased. When the report was released, Japanese doctors were interviewed on television to explain the high rate of smoking in Japan yet a low rate of lung cancer by stating that during World War II cigarettes were hard to obtain in Japan. However, the book *International Smoking Statistics*[98] gives figures for annual cigarette consumption for Japan for every year between 1920 and 1990, thus including World War Two. The figures in the book show that during the war there was a switch from standard cigarettes to hand rolled cigarettes, something the authors of the report did not take into account. The Japanese consumed 71,158 million cigarettes (a figure encompassing both roll-ups and standard) in 1941. The consumption rate stayed the same until 1944, when it dropped to 64,280 million cigarettes, at which time it rose until 1950 to 75,138 million cigarettes. Thus, whilst there was a dip in consumption, it was only for five years – at the end of, and after, the war – and nowhere near the extent to which Wynder would have us believe – from 71,158 million to 64,280 million, so not the third of the pre-war smoking rate that the report told us.

As with Doll, the most damaging (albeit overlooked) point is that Wynder himself admitted the data did not support smoking as a cause of lung cancer in Japan, as will be shown shortly. However, they also state that, of cancer of the larynx:

> The age adjusted mortality rates for laryngeal cancer during 1955 are higher in US White[s] than in the Japanese. These

---

[98] *International Smoking Statistics* (1993) Oxford University Press

differences can be partially explained by the higher levels of cigarette and alcohol consumption in the US.

and, of cancer of the oesophagus:

> In spite of the higher tobacco and alcohol consumption in the US, Japanese males have higher esophageal cancer mortality rates, which suggests that other risk factors are of importance.

Two things need mentioning here. Firstly, the researchers speak of a higher consumption of tobacco in Americans yet their own data shows the Japanese smoke more than the Americans. Secondly, they claim higher tobacco consumption rates of the US as a reason for higher rates of laryngeal cancer, yet when it comes to the Japanese having higher rates of oesophageal cancer despite smoking less they point out other factors are relevant. This is a classic case of twisting data to suit oneself. The only accurate thing to come from this is the acknowledgement of the truth that it is a ridiculous notion that smoking is the sole cause, or even major cause, of cancers of the larynx and oesophagus, and it is high time other factors were explored.

At the end of the report, Wynder admits that the study failed to link smoking and lung cancer:

> [lung cancer rates are] higher in US White men than in Japanese men which is discrepant with the higher prevalence of cigarette smoking among Japanese males for the same period of time.

The truth emerges! A lower incidence of lung cancer occurred in the heavier smoking Japanese, and a higher incidence with the lighter smokers in the USA. No matter how the figures are dressed up or twisted, the fact remains that the study spectacularly failed to show an increased risk of disease through tobacco smoking.

Wynder and Graham's 1950 study[99] which purported to link bronchogenic carcinoma to smoking is considered a landmark study, but is rife with problems. One major problem is that we are told the:

---

[99] http://tobaccodocuments.org/lor/87660204-0213.html#images

results of this report have not been obtained from hospital records since we learned at the outset of our study that the routine records did not supply satisfactory answers to our questions. It was therefore decided to seek the desired information by special interviews. Six-hundred and thirty-four patients reported on in this paper have been personally interviewed, and in 33 cases we obtained the information by mailing a questionnaire. In the remaining 17 cases information for the questionnaire was obtained from a person who had been intimately acquainted with the patient throughout his adult life.

Apparently, Wynder and Graham had a pre-set conclusion in mind and hospital results did not support this. Instead, they moved to questionnaires. Questionnaires are not a reliable source of information as they are fully dependent on the questions asked, how they are asked, the respondents understanding of them and both their honesty and accurate recollection. True science they are not. There is also the discrepancy of what an 'intimate acquaintance' is, as the term lends itself to a partner, lover, or close friend. Of course, such people are renowned for inaccurate recollections and, given that the patients were ill, recall bias. A further problem is that, as stated in the analysis of Doll's London Hospital study, the vast majority of people in the 1950s were smokers. Therefore, the study is guaranteed to produce a link between smoking and illness; however, the people who did not develop lung disease were also most likely smokers. Interestingly, those who smoked less than one cigarette a day for twenty years were considered non-smokers, meaning that many of them were actually smokers. However, because of the way it was calculated, someone who smoked a few cigarettes each day except the weekend, or a weekend social smoker, would have been classified as smoking one or fewer per day and thus a non-smoker. This means that a person could smoke 364 cigarettes a year and be considered a non-smoker.

The report states that the genders were reported separately, to account for any variation of the sexes. However, there were 642 males and only forty females, so the results do not permit comparison.

The study papers do include the questionnaire, and it is incredibly underwhelming.

1) Have you ever had a lung disease? If so, state time, duration and site of disease.
2) Do you or did you ever smoke?
3) At what age did you begin to smoke?
4) At what age did you stop smoking?
5) How much tobacco did you average per day during the past 20 years of your smoking?        Cigarettes…Cigars…Pipes
6) Do you inhale the smoke?
7) Do you have a chronic cough which you attribute to your smoking, especially upon first smoking in the morning?
8) Do you smoke before or after breakfast?
9) Name the brand or brands, and dates, if any given brand has been smoked exclusively for more than five years
10) What kind of jobs have you held? Have you been exposed to dust or fumes while working there?
11) Have you ever been exposed to irritative dusts or fumes outside of your job? In particular have you ever used insecticide spray excessively? If so, state time and duration
12) How much alcohol do you or have you averaged per day? State time and duration in years
13) Where were you born and where have you lived most of your life? State the appropriate time span you have lived in a certain locality. Up to what grade did you attend school?
14) State the cause of death of your parents, and of brothers and sisters[100]

This questionnaire is riddled with problems. For example, question five is guaranteed an inaccurate answer, as no one can state how much tobacco they smoked per day over twenty years. Question six can have multiple answers, for instance some people may inhale occasionally and others often, so it is not exclusively always or never. Question seven is forcing patients to make a medical opinion and, given they are suffering from a lung disease and their smoking habits are being brought into play by a doctor, they most likely then associated the two and answered 'yes', that they do attribute a cough to smoking. Question ten is requiring estimates of dust and fume exposure, but not many people can answer that appropriately.

---

[100] The full questionnaire can be seen in Appendix 2 at the end of this book

Worse still, it is not stated whether they should answer in time exposure i.e. five days a week for two years, or in quantity exposure i.e. light or heavy fumes, or indeed a mixture of the two i.e. heavy fumes for three hours a day. Furthermore, no thought has been given to the fact that some patients will answer one way, others another, so the results are neither comparable nor quantifiable. Question twelve is equally problematic, as it does not allow for people who drink perhaps once a week or on special occasions only. In short, this study is not a valid way of determining the effects of tobacco.

Nonetheless, despite Wynder and Graham conducting an incredibly flawed and bias study, they still do not say smoking is a cause of lung cancer. Instead, they conclude that they are tempted to say heavy smoking is a factor:

> it is apparent that smoking cannot be the only etiologic factor in the induction of the disease. From the evidence presented, however, the temptation is strong to incriminate excessive smoking, and in particular cigaret [sic] smoking, over a long period as at least one important factor

Even this study, riddled with problems and almost guaranteed to demonise smoking, found that there are other causes. Reading the study in detail, though, leads to the conclusion that had it been conducted without the use of a questionnaire and took a fair, objective look at tobacco use and lifestyle choice, tobacco would not be seen as increasing the rates of lung cancer. However, it is striking to note that even though Wynder and Graham blame smoking as a factor (rather than causative agent), they are keen to point out that it is heavy smoking over many years that they see as a problem, unlike today where we are told even light smokers have an elevated risk.

Norwegian Study Examining Health Consequences of Smoking

In late 2005 a new study was mentioned in the British news. The study was carried out in Norway and showed smoking just one to four cigarettes a day increased the risk of disease.[101] At first glance, the study looks to be well carried out: it has a relatively broad

---

[101] http://tobaccocontrol.bmj.com/cgi/content/full/14/5/315

population, covering Oslo and three other Norwegian counties, and a large population sample of 23,521 men and 19,201 women. The participants were screened for cardiovascular disease in the mid 1970s and followed until 2002. The outcome was absolute mortality and relative risks, adjusted for confounding variables, of dying from ischemic heart disease, all cancer, lung cancer, and from all causes. The results were:

> Adjusted relative risk (95% confidence interval) in smokers of 1-4 cigarettes per day, with never smokers as reference, of dying from ischaemic heart disease was 2.74 (2.07 to 3.61) in men and 2.94 (1.75 to 4.95) in women. The corresponding figures for all cancer were 1.08 (0.78 to 1.49) and 1.14 (0.84 to 1.55), for lung cancer 2.79 (0.94 to 8.28) and 5.03 (1.81 to 13.98), and for any cause 1.57 (1.33 to 1.85) and 1.47 (1.19 to 1.82).

The study also found the following:

> In men and women smoking 1-4 cigarettes per day, there was a distinct increase in risk of death from ischemic heart disease and from all causes. For ischemic heart disease, the steepest increase was in both sexes between 0 and 1-4 cigarettes per day. Above this level, the slope was less pronounced.

> For all disease groups and cigarette consumption levels, women had distinctly lower deaths rates than men; for ischemic heart disease women's risks related to never smokers, however, were clearly higher than in men. The same applies to risk for lung cancer in women smoking fewer than 20 cigarettes per day.
> It may be argued that the participants' smoking habits could have changed essentially since the screening took place. For example, analyses of results from the first screening indicate a steady increase in consumption during the first 10-20 years after starting to smoke. This may well have been the case, since the light smokers in this study had a shorter history of smoking than the other consumption groups. On the other hand, the light smokers may represent

previous heavier smokers who have cut down on consumption.

Some participants who were never smokers at baseline reported 10 years later that they were smokers, and this biases the relative risk estimate towards the null. On the other hand, a large proportion of light smokers had changed smoking category, but almost as many had quit smoking as had increased their consumption. The result of these changes is hard to quantify. It may even differ for the specific causes, as the dose-response relationship varies between them. In all, we see no strong reason to believe that the relative risk estimates for light smokers are substantially biased.

The quote "the result of these changes is hard to quantify" immediately raises suspicions of how reliable the results are, as it means they are largely at the mercy of how the researcher's want to interpret them.

We are told that cigarettes have most effect at one to four a day for ischemic heart disease, and after that the slope is less pronounced. Whilst they have recognised the slope goes down, apparently the slope does not level out after four cigarettes a day, meaning that whilst it has decreased slightly it still increases overall. If the risk still increases with each cigarette and one to four cigarettes pose so much threat, we could surely expect a very high rate of ischemic heart disease amongst smokers who smoke over a pack a day. However, this is not the case. In fact, ischemic heart disease is not recognised as a huge danger of smoking; of course, we are told that smoking increases the risk of heart disease, but it still plays second fiddle to cancer and probably emphysema and other respiratory illnesses. Yet, if even one to four cigarettes a day increase the risk of ischemic heart disease, it seems that, without a doubt, there would be an epidemic of it globally given the large percentages of people who smoke – 82% of British men in the 1950s, and 68% in America in the '60s. Even today, a quarter of the British population smoke. The fact is that the risk of ischemic heart disease apparently lowered after four cigarettes were smoked, which means that people on fifteen a day were only at a slightly increased risk over those smoking three a day. Thus, it is much more probable that the initial rise is the result of another factor that was not considered, such as exercise levels, diet or stress.

The researchers point out a flaw in the study themselves – the smoking habits of the participants changed. Any change in smoking habit will affect the results as it means that each category (i.e. how many cigarettes are smoked a day) is not measured individually, instead the participants change between categories. Such inconsistency drastically alters the results and it is impossible to effectively and accurately measure the risk of each category; if someone smoked heavily for twenty years then cut down, any effects from heavy smoking would be blamed on light smoking.

Another problem with the study is that the researchers say it was "adjusted for confounding variables", yet we are not told how these adjustments were made. Whilst it is possible that the researchers remained entirely objective and the adjustments were fair and valid, it is unlikely. If this is the case, I ask the question 'then why can't we see the adjustments?' After all, any researcher will want all their work on display for all to see, to prevent people saying they are withholding information that will invalidate the study. Apparently, though, these particular researchers felt it necessary to withhold the adjustments they made. I could conduct a study to prove anything, if I was allowed to adjust it any way I liked. Furthermore, to quote Lauren Colby again:

> Adjusting data is an invitation to bias or even outright fraud. If the smokers' life spans were significantly shorter than those of the never smokers, there shouldn't be any need to do any adjusting. The results should speak for themselves.

Clearly, then, these results did not speak for themselves – if they had, no adjustment would have been necessary.

Table two of the study shows the raw data, and table three shows the adjusted results. One thing the study did not account for was social class or overall lifestyle of the participants. The study also does not account for the genes of the participants, meaning that the fact they smoke may have been incidental if they have a predisposition to get a particular disease anyway.

Actually, I contacted the researchers with a query I had on the study, which they responded to. However, I then tried contacting them again to ask how they had singled out smoking as the factor responsible for the increased likelihood of disease, as they had failed to account for exercise levels, diet, genetics, and social status. Curiously, I received no reply for this question, again leaving me thinking they have something to hide with their findings.

Finally, another reason the study may have found a higher incidence of lung cancer in smokers is because of detection bias. The idea that smokers are so much more likely to get lung cancer than non-smokers is so entrenched within our society that people almost refuse to believe when non-smokers get it.

To conclude on this study, then, the results are incredibly underwhelming. The flawed methodology and apparent bias set the study up to have one outcome. In doing so, the researchers instantly rendered the study invalid as the results, and subsequent conclusion, are not born from objective research but a clear set agenda.

Native Americans and Smoking

The Native Americans are a very important part of discussion when looking at smoking and lung cancer, as they smoke and drink more than the average American. Tobacco has been a big part of their lives for longer than records have existed, and communal smoking of a sacred tobacco pipe remains a common ritual of many tribes. It was even considered a sacred part of their religion since they believed the smoke carried prayers to heaven. Tobacco is still used by them for its medicinal purposes.[102]

According to Centers for Disease Control and Prevention (CDC) in 2004, among youths, American Indian/Alaska Natives had the greatest cigarette smoking prevalence (23.1%), followed by non-Hispanic whites (14.9%), Hispanics (9.3%), non-Hispanic blacks (6.5%), and Asians (4.3%).[103]

A 2003 study, *Smoking Behavior Among Urban and Rural Native American Adolescents in California*[104] found that Native Americans had a "32% excess risk of past-month smoking compared with other groups". In addition, the smoking prevalence rates for those in urban and rural areas were almost exactly the same, at 27.7% and 29.3% respectively. Apparently, Native Americans reported "higher

---

[102] U.S. Department of Health and Human Services

[103] Centers for Disease Control and Prevention. Racial/Ethnic Differences Among Youths in Cigarette Smoking and Susceptibility to Start Smoking – United States, 2002-2004; Morbidity and Mortality Weekly Report. December 1, 2006; 55(47):1275-7

[104]http://www.ncbi.nlm.nih.gov/pubmed/14507533

access to cigarettes and exposure to smoking peers than other groups."

This data shows that Native Americans smoke more than the other ethnic divisions of America, including Hispanics and Caucasians. The life expectancy of Native American's is sixty-five, about thirteen years lower than America's average.[105] This does not appear to be from smoking-related diseases, though, rather the Native Americans have deaths from alcohol at six and a half times higher than the general population[106] and suicide rates are double those of the national average.[107] The Native Americans do suffer from lung cancer and other respiratory illnesses, which is to be expected, but the rates appear to be much lower than for the rest of the population. There have been two studies dealing with lung cancer amongst Native Americans, which are very interesting.

The first was conducted by J.M. Samet et al, of the University of New Mexico School of Medicine and published *Am J Public Health* in September 1988. Caucasians, Hispanics and Native Americans were looked at and the authors concluded that, for the study period of 1958 to 1982:

> [in whites] age adjusted mortality rates from lung cancer and from chronic obstructive pulmonary disease increased progressively in males and females. Mortality rates for both diseases increased in Hispanics during the study period, but the most recent rates for Hispanics were well below those for Other Whites...in Native Americans, rates for both diseases were low throughout the study period, and did not show consistent temporal trends.

Thus, the study concluded that whilst death rates from lung cancer and COPD increased in Hispanics during the study period it still remained much lower than for the rest of the general population. It must also be noted that, given the length of the study, medical advancements had been made and diagnosis improved, so increased

---

[105] National Indian Council on Aging, 1981

[106] Westermeyer, J.J. (1972). *Options regarding alcohol use among the Chippewa.* American Journal of Orthopsychiatry, 42, 398-403

[107] Shore, J.H. (1988). *Introduction. American Indian and Alaska Native Mental Health Research 1,* 3-4.

disease rates would be inevitable. Regarding Native Americans, the rates of both diseases remained low. In both cases, then, smoking appeared to have had no bearing on lung cancer or chronic obstructive pulmonary disease (COPD).

The second study was conducted by M.C. Mahoney et al, of the New York State Department of Health, using data from Native Americans in upstate New York between 1980 and 1986. It was published in the *International Journal of Epidemiology* in June 1989. Like the above study, this one had results that go against the typical view that smoking causes cancer, and discovered that the main causes of death amongst Native Americans were tuberculosis, diabetes, pneumonia and cirrhosis, and the researchers stated:

> fewer than expected malignant deaths occurred among both Native males and females...A deficit of deaths was observed for colon and lung cancer deaths among Native males and for colon and breast cancer deaths among Native females...

Malignant, of course, is another term for cancer, thus this quote breaks down as saying that higher rates of cancer were expected but they did not occur. There were lower rates of colon cancer deaths for both genders, and lower rates of lung and breast cancer deaths for men and women respectively than expected.

Thus, what transpires from these studies is that Native Americans smoke considerably more than the general population of the United States and yet suffer far less cancer – especially lung cancer. Given their high rates of diabetes, pneumonia, cirrhosis and tuberculosis, this low rate of cancer cannot simply be a result of healthy living or improved diet, and so there is no argument of their healthier living cancels out the negative effects of smoking.

The Nazi Discovery of Smoking and Cancer

When people state that the anti-smoking crusade is reminiscent of the Nazis, they are actually very accurate. Despite most people being ignorant to it, the Nazis coined the term 'passive smoking', implemented smoking bans and launched an attack on the habit. Nazis and smoking will be explored much more in chapter fourteen, but for now we will just look at how they 'discovered' that smoking causes cancer.

History often repeats itself, and at the time of writing there is a seemingly endless barrage of new anti-smoking studies. This is not unexpected, as the more 'evidence' the Tobacco Control movement collects the stronger it becomes. However, as we can see from looking at Germany around the time of World War Two, these studies are simply produced at the appropriate time and have very little scientific bearing. They are conducted and released to further instil the idea that smoking tobacco causes lung cancer, rather than an actual valid study showing a causative effect.

The first example of this is a publication from 1939 whereby Fritz Lickint, in collaboration with the Reich Committee for the Struggle against Addictive Drugs and the German Anti-Tobacco League, published *Tabak und Organismus* (*Tobacco and the Organism*). Professor Robert Proctor, who will be looked at later in this chapter, called the publication "arguably the most comprehensive scholarly indictment of tobacco ever published" and it found smoking tobacco was responsible for cancers of the lips, tongue, mouth, jaw, oesophagus, windpipe and lungs, as well as showing a "convincing argument" that passive smoking poses a threat to non-smokers.

It has been explained from the outset of this book how anti-smoking organisations fund studies to find smoking as harmful. This is no exception, and we see that it was conducted in collaboration with the German Anti-Tobacco League and the Reich Committee against drugs. Instantly this undermines the validity of the publication, as Hitler wanted a smoke-free Germany and, obviously, so did the anti-tobacco league.

In the late 1990s the United States had a series of articles and television documentaries which explained how the Nazis waged a war against smoking. Actually, the Nazis were known and admired for implementing the most progressive health policies of their time. Besides smoking, cancer was declared "number one enemy of the state" in Nazi Germany and they opposed sugar, fat, alcohol and sedentary lifestyles. Hitler himself was a vegetarian and avid anti-smoker.

The Nazis restricted smoking advertisements and implemented bans in many workplaces and government offices, hospitals, and all city trains and buses. In addition to this, women were not allowed to buy cigarettes, by law, in certain places, with one slogan exclaiming "The German woman does not smoke".

Professor Robert Proctor wrote a book entitled *The Nazi War on Cancer*,[108] in which he praised the Nazis for realising how fatal smoking is. On page 194, Proctor mentions what he calls "an exquisite piece of scholarship", a study conducted by Hans Muller in 1939 which 'proved' smoking causes lung cancer. Until that point in the book, Proctor had mentioned little to nothing in the way of scientific support despite praising the Nazi organisation for discovering smoking is deadly. However, apparently that is of little consequence as Muller's study was so definitive that no further proof was needed. As usual, though, things are not what they seem.

Muller's study was a retrospective study, whereby he sent a questionnaire to the relatives of people who died from lung cancer. The questionnaire is as follows:

1. Was the deceased Herr ___ a smoker? If so, what his daily consumption of cigars, cigarettes, or pipe tobacco? Please be numerically precise in your answer!
2. Did the deceased smoke at some point in his life and then stop? Until when did he smoke? If he did smoke, what was his daily consumption of cigars, cigarettes or pipe tobacco? (Please be precise!)
3. Did the deceased ever cut down on his smoking? How high was his daily use of tobacco products, before and after he cut back? (Please be precise!)
4. Can you say whether the deceased was ever exposed to polluted air for any length of time, either at work or off the job? Did this unclean air contain smoke, soot, dust, tar, fumes, motor exhaust, coal dust or metallic dust, industrial chemicals, cigarette smoke, or similar substances?

First things first, the questions themselves are very direct and focus specifically on smoking without any regard to other factors except for question four. However, that question is dependent on the recipient knowing what contaminants were present in the air, something that is highly unlikely if not impossible, and does not account for how long the deceased was exposed to it, for how many days, weeks or years etc. and in what concentrations the asked contaminants were. Muller did not ask seemingly obvious, not to mention necessary, questions such as what profession the deceased

---

[108] Proctor, R. N. (1999) *The Nazi War on Cancer* Princeton University Press

had, what his lifestyle in terms of exercise, diet or alcohol intake was, or whether there was a genetic history of cancer in the family. It is all well and good asking the questions he did, but they are meaningless without other data. Plus, if the majority of the population smoked then the majority of lung cancer victims will be smokers – and the majority were, indeed, smokers.

The problems with retrospective studies have already been explained i.e. that they are dependent on the person being questioned having a good memory, and the results are invariably skewed by recall bias e.g. if a person dies of lung cancer and smoked then the person being questioned is likely to exaggerate the amount the deceased smoked, for two reasons: firstly, they are being forced to remember them smoking, and secondly, the deceased died of lung cancer and so the interviewee will automatically think 'he must have smoked a lot or he would not have developed cancer'. This is well known to psychologists, it is a combination of faith in researchers and the fact that leading questions can shape the recipient's answer. Put another way, the more questions regarding health effects of smoking the recipient has to answer, the more they will make a link between smoking and disease.

The next problem with the 'study' is that Muller does not say how many questionnaires were sent out, but we are told that ninety-six were obtained. This is an identical methodology to Doll's British Doctor's study, whereby the results were tainted by self-selecting participants. The problem with this is that it is possible many people decided to take part because their relative(s) had died from lung cancer. This is an issue that would have been eradicated had Muller used a cross-selection of participants. Besides Muller only having ninety-six participants, which is in itself a low population sample, we also do not know how close that number is to the number of questionnaires sent out. For instance, for all we know, there could have been 1,000 questionnaires sent out, meaning those ninety-six are less than a tenth of what could have been obtained. Muller's refusal to say how many were sent out could indicate it was quite a high number.

A further problem arrives when we see that, of those ninety-six participants, eighty-six were male and only ten were female. There is a large imbalance between genders, and ten females is far too small a sample to be able to gather any scientific information.

The eighty-six males were divided into five groups: extremely heavy smoker, very heavy smoker, heavy smoker, moderate smoker, or non-smoker. Muller then obtained eighty-six controls (the controls being smokers without cancer) of the same age as the participants to compare the lung cancer rates between the groups. Proctor informs us that Muller found that the lung cancer victims were over six times as likely to be extremely heavy smokers as the controls. 16% of the healthy group were non-smokers, compared to 3.5% of the lung cancer victims. Apparently the lung cancer victims smoked a total of 2,900 grams of tobacco per day, whilst the healthy controls smoked 1,250 grams per day (again, early research shows light smoking as being innocent regarding the onset of disease). It has to be said, though, that it is quite puzzling that both the controls and study groups were smokers as there is then nothing to compare. For instance, if group A were smokers and group B non-smokers, then comparisons can be made. However, if groups A and B are both smokers, or partly consist of smokers, then no conclusion can be drawn because smoking has not been made an isolated factor.

Whether Muller intentionally withheld information or whether he did not feel it necessary is not known, although when a study is carried out correctly researchers cannot spell out the methodology fast enough, as it prevents backlash, criticisms of bias, and faulty work etc. The fact is he left us to guess a lot. We do not know how Muller selected either the cancer victims or the controls, so the study is wide open to the criticism that he was free to pick and choose the ones that backed up his hypothesis that smoking causes lung cancer. On top of this, he was able to choose the controls on any criteria he wanted; for example, he could have chosen smokers who ate well and lived stress free lives, or without a genetic predisposition to cancer, and so on. By carefully selecting his controls, he was able to minimise the chance of his results disproving his hypothesis.

Perhaps the most damaging problem is that Muller compared the recollections of living smokers with relatives of deceased smokers. A smoker is able to say with much more accuracy how much they smoke on a day-to-day basis than a relative of a smoker who died years previously. A relative, for example, would not be around the deceased smoker every waking moment, so cannot possibly estimate a number of cigarettes smoked. Thus, the results are incomparable.

There have been many studies on people and conformity – Nazism itself is an often used topic in Psychology when discussing conformity – and any psychologist will explain that the majority of people will conform to the trend or bow down to authority figures. As such, this next issue is very important and cannot be overstated. As has been observed already regarding retrospective studies, there is a tendency for those being asked to recollect their relatives' smoking habits to exaggerate the number unwittingly, especially as during 1930s Germany there was a very strong anti-smoking campaign going on. However, there was a reverse bias for the healthy controls. In Germany at the time, as part of the anti-smoking campaign, propaganda minister Goebbels was saturating the German press with articles suggesting that smokers were almost as bad as Jews, and generally out-casting smokers in a bid to eradicate smoking, or at least minimise it. Because of the way smoking was viewed at the time, when the controls were asked how much they smoked it was typical for them to state they smoked much less than they actually did in order to appear to be better citizens or appear to not be 'full-blown' smokers – meaning they may well have smoked as much as those with cancer.

At the end of the book Proctor offered figures provided by the American Cancer Society and Krebsforschungszentrum, the German Cancer Research Centre. The figures show that in West Germany in 1952 the LCDR was twenty-two per 100,000 population in men and four for women, compared to twenty-five per 100,000 for American men and five for American women. In 1990, the German rates were forty-nine and eight for men and women respectively, and thirty-five and thirty-two for men and women respectively in America. We are then told the figures are age adjusted, but we are not told how. It is claimed that the American LCDRs went much higher than those of the Germans because of the delayed effect of the German smoking ban, which translates to a delayed effect of smoking to twenty-five to forty-five years. Because during and after World War Two women were practically forbidden to smoke and tobacco was very hard to obtain, there should have been a significant lowering of disease and increase in life expectancy anywhere between 1964 and 1990. However, this is not the case. A 1987 database states that West German women had a life expectancy of seventy-eight, whereas women in the USA had a life expectancy of seventy-nine. The German men and American men had life expectancies of seventy-one and seventy-two respectively; meaning German men and women had lower life-expectancies than the Americans. By comparison, Switzerland had a life expectancy in the database of 80 for women and seventy-three for men, higher than both the Germans and Americans even though their smoking habits were unaffected during the war. Even today, Switzerland has a life expectancy of over eighty, whereas Germany's is just over seventy-four, so the incubation theory fails to show why the German life expectancy did not exceed that of Switzerland despite the former consuming much less tobacco.

Thus, we should learn from history, as well as our past examples and mistakes, to realise that this current war on smoking is ridiculous and unfounded – Germany had no increased life expectancy or healthier citizens as a result of their smoking bans or reduced consumption. The fact that they had lower life expectancies of both those in the USA and Switzerland should really tell us that neither smoking nor its cessation has any bearing on life expectancy.

## Have Researchers Discovered How Tobacco Smoking Causes Cancer?

In October 1996, researchers claimed they had found the exact mechanism of how smoking causes cancer. The study, *Preferential Formation of Benzo[a]pyrene Adducts at Lung Cancer Mutational Hotspots in P53,* was published in *Science* magazine.[109] As one can imagine, it was considered a massive breakthrough because, if the study was correct, there would be irrefutable proof that tobacco smoking causes cancer. Not only that, they could prove *how* it does. Some people, even in health authorities, still use the study to show we have proof smoking is deadly. However, in keeping with the familiar theme of smoking studies, this one is of no validity and does nothing to show if, or how, cigarette smoking is harmful. The first thing we are told is:

> Cigarette smoke carcinogens such as benzo[a]pyrene are implicated in the development of lung cancer. The distribution of benzo[a]pyrene diol epoxide (BPDE) adducts along exons of the P53 gene in BPDE-treated HeLa cells and bronchial epithelial cells was mapped at nucleotide resolution. Strong and selective adduct formation

---

[109] http://www.sciencemag.org/cgi/content/abstract/274/5286/430

occurred at guanine positions in codons 157, 248, and 273. These same positions are the major mutational hotspots in human lung cancers. Thus, targeted adduct formation rather than phenotypic selection appears to shape the P53 mutational spectrum in lung cancer. These results provide a direct etiological link between a defined chemical carcinogen and human cancer.

The truth is in there somewhere, but it is not what is presented. It is true that Benzo[a]pyrene (BAP) has been linked to cancer (but is a possible human carcinogen, not a known human carcinogen), and it is true that BAP is in cigarette smoke. However, it is *not* true that the amount of BAP present in smoke is nearly enough to lead to the onset of disease. As explained in chapter two, the richest source of BAP is leafy green vegetables, where they pick it up from the surrounding air. So, then, if the researchers are telling us the BAP in cigarette smoke is responsible for lung cancer, they are also telling us (or should be telling us) that green vegetables and outside air is responsible. For some reason, though, they are not mentioning that. Moreover, they used an isolated chemical, rather than tobacco smoke itself. They are unable therefore to claim smoking causes cancer because there may well be other chemicals in the smoke that negate the damage; for instance it is a known fact that anti-carcinogens are present in tobacco smoke.

The study claims that damage to the p53 gene in lung cancer incidences of smokers proves that cigarette smoking damages the gene, thus leading to the onset of lung cancer. Somehow, though, the researchers ignored the fact that they not only could not prove it, but defeated their own argument straight away. They start off by saying that there is damage to the p53 "guardian angel" gene – so-called because some believe it protects against cancer – in roughly 60% of lung cancer cases. The problem here is that this means in 40% of lung cancer cases there is no damage to the gene. This means that in almost half of the cases, the p53 gene is undamaged; therefore lung cancer can be contracted regardless of the condition of the gene. Lung cancer exists in its victims regardless of their p53 gene being damaged or not, and as such it is impossible to claim cigarette smoke causes lung cancer through damage to the gene. There is also the realisation that the researchers did not actually study any human lung cancers. Instead of human lung cancers, they looked at cultured human cells which they exposed to a "metabolite" of BAP, known as Benzo[a]pyrene diolepoxide (BAPDE). The researchers then tested the cells for mutational damage and said they found mutations at certain locations on the genes, similar to those in 60% of lung cancer cases. It is imperative to look closely at the language used, because a subtle word change can make the difference between something and nothing. They claimed that the mutations were *similar* to those in 60% of lung cancer cases, but they did not say *identical*. It would be interesting to see in what regard they were similar, as that could mean anything from size to location.

Let us take a second look: the researchers have already said p53 gene damage is not present in all lung cancers; they did not study real human lung cancers when exposing lungs to BAP; and they exposed cultured human cells to a metabolite of BAP. A metabolite is, according to definition, "a substance produced by metabolism". Metabolism takes place in the gut and the liver, and the products flow into the bloodstream where they reach the lungs during the process of re-oxygenation. As mentioned in chapter two, BAP is found in lots of places in higher concentrations than smoke, and studies have shown that over 90% of the BAP consumed by humans, including smokers, comes from food. It is the authors' claim that in order for BAP to become carcinogenic it must be converted to BAPDE, but this causes two problems. Firstly, the amount of BAP reaching the lungs in the blood supply, which is metabolised to BAPDE elsewhere in the body, would far exceed the amount present in cigarette smoke. Secondly, there is no evidence anywhere to suggest that the lungs can metabolise BAP into BAPDE. In order for this study to be correct, the lungs would need to metabolise BAP to BAPDE, as in this way smokers would receive significantly more BAPDE than non-smokers.

We are then told that, given the researchers had no humans to work with, the mutations which they had induced were compared with specimens of DNA taken from a gene database that had been compiled by others. What would be logical, expected and scientifically necessary, would be for the researchers to compare the genes of smokers with lung cancer with non-smokers who have lung cancer to see if there is a difference in the tumours. This would, after all, eradicate all doubt that there is no evidence smoking causes an individual case of lung cancer, as it would show conclusively whether specific incidences of cancer were caused by smoking or not. Alas, they did not do this. In fact, the researchers deliberately excluded any DNA samples obtained from non-smokers or from "radon associated cancers". Interestingly enough, they did not tell us how they knew whether any particular samples came from non-smokers or were 'radon associated'; it appears they took the word of the people who compiled the database. Regardless, the fact is that experiments are meant to be controlled, yet these researchers dismissed the controls that would skew their results.

Finally, we are told that "This study provides a direct link between a defined cigarette smoke carcinogen and human cancer mutations." However, this study failed to show that because they were looking specifically at BAPDE and not BAP itself. As there is no BAPDE in cigarette smoke and there is no evidence to show the lungs can metabolise BAP to BAPDE, this claim cannot be made. The researchers also cannot claim to have found an indirect link as people get most of their BAP exposure from food, and an indirect link would mean that what we eat can cause lung cancer. The study does not account for the 40% of lung cancer victims who do not have damage to their p53 gene, which suggests that the gene is irrelevant to the development or presence of cancer. Moreover, the researchers compared their results with DNA samples which they selectively picked, rather than random selection or comparing with all the data available. This means, of course, that they selectively chose the samples which would prove their hypothesis.

In short, the study does not prove anything. The researchers failed to prove their claim and it does not take much critical analysis of the study to see how flawed it is. The fact the article got published and is regularly cited and praised speaks volumes about the current view of smoking. That an inaccurate, misleading and misinformative article can get published means that it is being done so because it is against smoking; any other subject would have either been critically reviewed beforehand, or been critically assessed in the same edition of the magazine. This study was seemingly subjected to neither.

## World Data

One of the most damaging counter arguments to the anti-smokers claim that smoking will kill people is the data for the rest of the world. If, as we are led to believe, smoking will lead to disease and a decreased life expectancy, then why is it that the countries with the highest rates of smokers also have the longest life expectancy? It cannot be solely down to the medical advances, as no country in the world has a conventional medical system that cures cancer. As a matter of fact, the success rate of conventional medicine on cancer is very low – lung cancer only has a five-year success rate of about 7%. [110]

Japan has one of the longest life expectancies in the world, at seventy-eight for men and eighty-five for women, yet the Japanese also have one of the highest rates of smokers in the world at over 33%. In the United Kingdom and the USA smoking rates have been declining for years, yet the rates of cancer have been increasing.

Consider these statistics from the 1990s, compiled by the WHO and the CIA:

Top 15 Male Life Expectancies (LE):

| Country | LE (years) | Smokers prevalence (%) |
|---|---|---|
| 1. Iceland | 76.6 (1994) | 31.0 (1994) |
| 2. Japan | 76.5 (1994) | 59.0 (1994) |
| 3. Costa Rica | 75.9 (1994) | 35.0 (1988) |
| 4. Israel | 75.9 (1994) | 45.0 (1990) |
| 5. Sweden | 75.5 (1994) | 22.0 (1994) |
| 6. Greece | 75.2 (1994) | 46.0 (1994) |
| 7. Switzerland | 74.8 (1994) | 36.0 (1992) |
| 8. Netherlands | 74.7 (1994) | 36.0 (1994) |
| 9. Canada | 74.7 (1994) | 31.0 (1991) |
| 10. Cuba | 74.7 (1994) | 49.3 (1990) |
| 11. Australia | 74.5 (1994) | 29.0 (1993) |

[110] http://info.cancerresearchuk.org/cancerstats/types/lung/

| 12. | Spain | 74.5 (1994) | 48.0 (1993) |
| 13. | Malta | 74.5 (1994) | 40.0 (1992) |
| 14. | Italy | 74.4 (1994) | 38.0 (1994) |
| 15. | France | 74.3 (1994) | 40.0 (1993) |
| | USA | 72.6 (1994) | 28.1 (1991) |

Figures from 2002-2003 show the smoking consumption of 30 countries:[111] [112]

| Country | Smoking Prevalence (%) | LE |
| --- | --- | --- |
| Austria | 36.3 | 78.6 |
| Greece | 35 | 78.1 |
| Hungary | 33.8 | 72.4 |
| Luxembourg | 33 | 78.2 |
| Turkey | 32.1 | 68.7 |
| Netherlands | 32 | 78.6 |
| South Korea | 30.4 | 77.5 |
| Japan | 30.3 | 81.8 |
| Spain | 28.1 | 80.5 |
| Denmark | 28 | 77.2 |
| Poland | 27.6 | 74.7 |
| Belgium | 27 | 78.1 |
| Ireland | 27 | 77.8 |
| France | 27 | 79.4 |
| Switzerland | 26.8 | 80.4 |
| Mexico | 26.4 | 74.9 |
| Norway | 26 | 79.5 |
| UK | 26 | 78.5 |
| New Zealand | 25 | 78.7 |

---

[111] http://www.nationmaster.com/graph/hea_dai_smo-health-daily-smokers

[112] http://www.swivel.com/graphs/show/11973744 (S.Korea LE taken from http://www.highbeam.com/doc/1G1-139943100.html)

| | | |
|---|---|---|
| Germany | 24.3 | 78.4 |
| Slovakia | 24.3 | 73.9 |
| Italy | 24.2 | 79.9 |
| Czech Republic | 24.1 | 75.3 |
| Iceland | 22.4 | 80.7 |
| Finland | 22.2 | 78.5 |
| Portugal | 20.5 | 77.3 |
| Australia | 19.8 | 80.3 |
| Sweden | 17.5 | 80.2 |
| USA | 17.5 | 77.2 |
| Canada | 17 | 79.7 |

It would appear, then, that smoking has never led to a decrease in life expectancy or a decreased population. As a matter of fact, it seems that the establishment is being forced to take note of the fact that lung cancer still exists despite the decline in smokers. In 2007, 43% of lung cancer victims were non-smokers, compared to 57% who were smokers. In America, the lung cancer societies have run commercials featuring non-smokers who have suffered, or are suffering, from lung cancer, asking for research money.

This is interesting, given that in Britain we are still subjected to the same adverts only showing smokers afflicted with lung cancer or respiratory problems, leading the public to associate the two and forget that non-smokers also get these diseases. This is extremely damaging, as it prevents research going into the true cause and treatment of diseases, and leads the public into thinking if they don't smoke then they are unlikely to get disease. It is a curious point that many people fail to think food has much bearing on their overall health and wellbeing, despite foods now being destroyed by GM crops, pesticides, preservatives, artificial sweeteners and chemicals and poor quality food production.

There are official records of cigarette consumption for countries around the world and, as usual, the data does not support the notion that smoking kills, or causes lung cancer. The *Oxford Atlas of the World* from 1992 gives figures for cigarette consumption for 1986–1988. The figures are of annual consumption of cigarettes per capita.

| Country | Consumption |
|---|---|
| Hungary | 2515 |

| | |
|---|---|
| Japan | 2510 |
| USA | 2020 |
| South Africa | 1950 |
| UK | 1700 |
| France | 1690 |
| USSR | 1650 |
| Brazil | 1200 |
| Philippines | 1150 |
| Venezuala | 950 |
| Zaire | 150 |
| India | 100 |

These figures can be used in conjunction with the lung cancer death rates (LCDRs) for each country. The World Bank has a book giving statistics for a number of countries which give statistics of disease in a form of "45Q15". This number represents the percentage risk of someone who is fifteen years of age dying from a particular disease before they are sixty. Unfortunately, not all the countries in the above table are in the book, such as the USSR and India, however there are plenty of others and a few missing countries will not make any difference. The following statistics are in the 45Q15 format, meaning they are risk figures in percentages.

The male LCDR in the USA is 1.4%, and for females 0.7%. Hungary, with the highest rate of cigarette consumption in the world in 1992, had a LCDR of 2.4% for males and 0.5% for women. Japan, second in the list by a marginal amount, has a male LCDR of 0.5% (which works out to be about a fifth of the Hungarian rate and a third of the U.S. rate), and for females it is 0.3%. Finally, the World Bank inform us that the Chinese are a nation of smokers, and there is now much publicity into how much they are smoking and how their rates of smoking are increasing rapidly, yet their LCDR is roughly the same as that of the Japanese – 0.56% for men, and 0.59% for women.

It is obvious that there is more to the onset of lung cancer than smoking but it is impossible to pin down any single factor as the cause. Of course, some people may point out that it is misdiagnosis and poorer healthcare systems that are responsible for the low rates of lung cancer in these countries. This is, however, a fallacy. Japan has an exceptional healthcare system, and it would be impossible to have the longest life expectancy in the world by having poor healthcare and misdiagnosis as a regularity. Naturally, some countries do have such systems, but there are others with high smoking rates and good healthcare systems, such as Hungary. In Hungary there are no deaths attributed to 'ill defined' causes; meaning every death has a decided explanation. Japan has an 'ill defined' rate of only 0.1% for males and 0% for females, meaning the cases of lung cancer are always, or almost always, accounted for and diagnosed. China has a similar rate, with 'ill defined' rates for both men and women of less than 0.1%. What this means is that these countries not only have low levels of lung cancer, but that they also account for each death – meaning, positively, they genuinely have low rates of lung cancer, and not that they are overlooking the cases.

The most important thing is that the statistics do not waver, proving that the statistics of one year are not mere fluke. Let us look at the rates in 1994: at this time, Iceland had the highest life expectancy, of 76.6 years, and 31% of males smoked. Japan was second-highest with a life expectancy of 76.5 years, and 59% of the men smoked. Israel had a life expectancy of 75.9 and 45% of men smoked. Greece was not far behind, with a life expectancy of 75.2 and 46% smokers. Finally, Cuba and Spain had an expectancy of 74.7 and 74.5 respectively, and a smokers' prevalence of 49.3% and 48% respectively.

Further figures tell the following: in 1939, *Fortune* magazine reported that 53% of American adults males smoked, and 66% of males under forty years of age smoked; in 1900 4.4 billion cigarettes were sold; in 1901 3.5 billion cigarettes and six billion cigars were sold; the 1930 market share shows that 43.2 billion Lucky Strike were sold, 35.3 billion Camel were sold, and over thirty-five billion cigarettes sold across three other brands (Chesterfield, Old Gold, and Raleigh).

This tells us that the information we are bombarded with by anti-smokers is simply incorrect. The problem is, the figures are never challenged and as such they are never required to be validated or backed up. This is something that clearly has implications, as it gives those with the power to simply make figures up with no fear of repercussions or humiliation for being wrong. One thing we are told regularly is that smoking will rob smokers of ten years of their life (Mr. Van der Griendt states on his website that smoking reduces life expectancy by up to 25 years!), if what the anti-smoking organisations were saying was true, they would never let people have any doubt and would constantly present the relevant data.

The USA is very interesting with its smoking habits, and we can learn a lot merely from looking at them over the years. According to page fourteen of the 1964 Surgeon General's Report, cigarette consumption in America was fifty cigarettes per capita per annum in 1900; 138 in 1910; 1,965 in 1930; 1,828 in 1940, and 3,322 in 1950. In 1961 cigarette smoking peaked at 3,986, and in that year over half of men over eighteen years old were smokers.

Smoking rates then began to decline, as by 1964, when the Report came out, the American Cancer Society's campaign was having an effect and people were beginning to cease the habit, or less people were taking it up. Either way, according to the aforementioned figures from *Oxford Atlas of the World*, by 1986-1988 the consumption per capita per annum was down to 2,020. A Surgeon General's Report from 1980 reported that in 1965 51.1% of adult men smoked, and 33.3% of women. The same Report tells us that the figures in 1979 were 36.9% for men and 28.2% for women. The Centers for Disease Control (CDC) tells us that in 1992 just 26.5% of all Americans were smokers, and of these 22.1% were regular smokers and 4.4% were occasional smokers.

At this time, there were approximately 180 million Americans who were aged over eighteen. If we assume that the average amount smoked is a pack a day, then it is possible to get the annual per capita cigarette consumption by taking 26% of 180 million to get the number of smokers. This is fifty-one million. We then multiply that by 365 days (one year) to get the annual consumption of all fifty-one million smokers and dividing by 180 million to obtain the per capita annual consumption. This yields a result of 2,069 cigarettes per annum per capita, a number very close to the one given by the *Oxford Atlas* which gives 2,020. With this information, we can view America as one big experiment from which we can view the cigarette/lung cancer link.[113] Firstly, if 50% of smokers die from their habit then America would have lost ninety million people from its population – it didn't. Secondly, we should see a decrease in LCDR's between 1961 and 1992, since there was a decline in the rates of smoking and cigarette consumption. However, no such decrease in lung cancer has occurred. In fact, the opposite is true, and lung cancer rates have continued to rise despite lower rates of smoking.

We can see this in the statistics offered by the Statistical Abstract of the United States, published by the Commerce Department in 1993. The statistics show cancer death rates for men and women between 1970 and 1990. The figures are given as deaths per 100,000 of population, instead of percentages. Thus, when the figures refer to a particular age group, they refer to the number of deaths per 100,000 of the population in that particular age group, making the figures automatically age adjusted. What we can see from the following table (years 1970-1990) is that there are increases in every group except men aged 35-44, and that group has a low rate of cancer anyway. This is of no surprise, given that cancer is typically a disease of the elderly.

Men:

| A g e Group | 1 | 1980 | 1990 |
|---|---|---|---|
| 35-44 | 17.0 | 12.6 | 9.1 |
| 45-54 | 72.1 | 79.8 | 63.0 |
| 55-64 | 202.3 | 223.8 | 232.6 |
| 65-74 | 340.7 | 422.0 | 447.3 |
| 75-84 | 354.2 | 511.5 | 594.4 |
| 85 + | 215.3 | 386.3 | 538.0 |

Women:

---

[113] *In Defense of Smokers* www.lcolby.com

| A   g   e Group | 1970 | 1980 | 1990 |
|---|---|---|---|
| 35-44 | 6.5 | 6.8 | 5.4 |
| 45-54 | 22.2 | 34.8 | 35.3 |
| 55-64 | 38.9 | 74.5 | 107.6 |
| 65-74 | 45.6 | 106.1 | 181.7 |
| 75-84 | 56.5 | 98.0 | 194.5 |
| 85+ | 56.5 | 96.3 | 142.8 |

What is particularly interesting is that the cancer rates for women have increased much more dramatically than they have for men. The reason for this is unknown, it could be anything from increased diagnosis to chemicals in make-up; it is not my place to make a judgement on the reason. However, what is clear from these figures is that the lung cancer rates have risen steadily, whilst the rate of smoking has declined steadily. Apparently, though, according to the anti-smokers, smoking is still responsible for this rise in LCDR's. They have introduced something known as the "incubation theory", in which we are told that it takes twenty to thirty years for the effects of smoking to cause disease in the body, and as women apparently started smoking twenty to thirty years after men, this explains the discrepancy in the figures.

There are numerous problems with this theory, notwithstanding the fact that it is far too convenient that lung cancer rates rose for women the same number of years after they started smoking i.e. 20-30 years. This is simply too linear, given that not all smokers develop cancer and not all cancers occur at the same age.

Contrary to popular belief, women did not start smoking as late as we are led to believe. Bearing in mind cigarette smoking did not become really popular until after World War Two (1945), women were smoking about the same time as men. In 1944, a Gallup poll found that 36% of American women over seventeen years old were smokers.[114] The Department of Agriculture, in 1959, estimated that 47% of the overall population of the United States over the age of fourteen smoked, and that men smoked, on average, twenty-four cigarettes a day and women smoked nineteen a day.[115] Furthermore, let us not forget how iconic the cigarette was for women in 1920s art such as films and paintings. Leading ladies in popular films of the time were rarely seen without a cigarette in a cigarette holder. Subsequent surveys from between 1955 and 1985 cited in *International Smoking Statistics* show female smoking rates as being between 27% and 37%, with later surveys in 1985 at between 25% and 28%. What these figures serve to prove is that women were not latecomers into the field of smoking, and have been partaking in tobacco use for seemingly as long as men have. Certainly, there is no evidence to the contrary, and the anti-smoking organisations are not displaying any such information.

Another problem with the 'incubation' theory is that the statistics for LCDR's in women do not add up when compared with the overall cancer death rate in women i.e. the rate of death from cancers of all kinds, combined.[116] The Statistical Abstract informs us that the overall cancer death rate, age adjusted, has remained practically constant over the years, being 108.8 in 1970 and 112.7 in 1990. This seems to be a paradox given that the rate of LCDR's has dramatically increased in women. However, it is important to remember that we are talking about death rates and not just incidence of disease, and whilst lung cancer rates have increased, rates of other diseases have decreased. For example, the death rate in females from ischemic heart disease:

| Age Group | 1970 | 1980 | 1990 |
|-----------|-------|-------|-------|
| 45-54 | 84.0 | 52.2 | 33.6 |
| 55-64 | 299.1 | 164.5 | 135.4 |
| 65-74 | 978.0 | 430.1 | 415.2 |

---

[114] *International Smoking Statistics* (1993) Oxford University Press, ISBN 0 19 262485 7

[115] *Facts on File* 29th April 1959

[116] *In Defense of Smokers* www.lcolby.com

| 75-84 | 2866.3 | 1842.7 | 1287.6 |
| 85+ | 6951.5 | 5280.6 | 4257.8 |

We can see from those figures that the death rate from ischemic heart disease for females has fallen considerably. Furthermore, whilst the success rate of cancer is still very low and conventional medicine has by no means 'won the war', so to speak, the incidence of success is now better than it was, thanks in part to increased diagnosis and the subsequent ability to catch the disease in its early stages.

Finally, one particularly damaging point is that Dr. B.K.S. Dijkstra, of the University of Pretoria, showed during World War Two smoking rates fell to zero – simply because no tobacco was available.[117] However, during the same time frame the lung cancer rate neither fell nor stayed the same – it actually increased. Some people will try to counter this by bringing up the incubation theory. In fact, this is a huge problem with the anti-smokers – when history does not show lung cancer to be associated with smoking they invent a lag to make it fit. However, when they called for a ban the health benefits were to be immediate, such as heart attack admissions and so forth. The Cancer Research UK website even states that lung cancer rates have declined as a result of smoking rates declining – yet their own theory would dictate that our current level of lung cancer rates caused by smoking would be due to smoking rates in 1979! This raises another point: if smoking carries a thirty year incubation period but other factors do not (necessarily) how do we know whether the lung cancer rates of today are from something we improved or discovered recently, or something that happened in 1979?

It transpires that all the available data, going back many years, shows that smoking does not affect life expectancy. Clearly, there is no evidence that smoking will decrease the life of a person or a nation, and the decline of smoking rates has not resulted in a decline in lung cancer, leading to the conclusion that smoking has no bearing on either lung cancer or death. If it did, the results would speak for themselves, and the anti-smoking organisations would make sure those results were heard constantly. Instead,

---

[117] Dijkstra, B.K.S. *South African Cancer Bulletin* Vol. 21 No. 1

though, they merely give useless theories and false data knowing that it will remain unchallenged. When it is challenged, though, it does not hold up.

## Cancer and Genetics

At this point the book has shown that, to this day, we actually have no real evidence that smoking causes cancer. Everyone knows of an elderly smoker, and these are hardly exceptions – it is not uncommon to see an elderly person smoking, and typically they smoke quite heavily – and where else do we tend to see cigar and pipe smokers than in the elderly? Whilst there are an abundance of figures and quotes that the media constantly presents, there are actually far fewer studies than one would probably imagine and, as shown, they typically receive funding from anti-smoking organisations such as the American Cancer Society. Accordingly, they produce results which keep the sponsors happy However, a critical look at the studies shows that they leave a lot to be desired and fall very short of the mark – from skewed results and thrown out controls, all sorts of manipulative methods are employed to ensure a study yields the desired results.

As has also been shown, I am not the only person to be doubting the link between smoking and cancer. The following all feel that the link has either been grossly exaggerated for political reasons, or that there is no link at all: Lauren Colby, an American lawyer who wrote his own book on the topic, *In Defense of Smokers*; Philip Burch, whose thoughts have been mentioned regarding Doll's study of British Doctor's; Eysenck, who was briefly explained and will be again in a moment; and Dr. Whelan – an anti-smoker who we will explore in the following chapter – admits that there is no evidence to show second-hand smoke causes disease in non-smokers. There are, of course, many more that question or refute the smoking and lung cancer connection, and many of these people are well educated people such as doctors, lawyers, scientists, or researchers themselves.

Something else that has been shown is the agendas and bias present in anti-smoking studies, and it says a lot that these agendas exist to begin with. Furthermore, some researchers have even stated their study/studies are/were fraudulent or did not show what they were claimed to show, such as Doll and Wynder. Given this, why are we still expected to believe smoking causes lung cancer? Given that the researchers trying to prove the link fail to do so, that no animal study has ever managed to succeed, and that world data shows the opposite, perhaps it is time this notion was challenged and discarded. The research has been done, no credible evidence has been found, so, as real science should do and does elsewhere, we should move on. So why do we not?

The answer to that is most likely because of the question it would inevitably lead to: 'then what does cause lung cancer?' As was said in the Introduction, the ACS conducted a very early study to blame cancer on smoking as they were frustrated with not knowing what caused the disease. Sadly, conventional medicine has not really moved on much and we still have no cure for the disease. There are many alternative therapies, which have very high success rates (such as Laetrile, the Budwig Diet and others), yet they, unsurprisingly, fall under the scrutiny of the great Health Establishment which demonises smoking – where at best the therapy is ignored, overlooked or hidden, and at worst the scientist behind it is thrown in prison, as happened to Ryke Geerd Hamer. However, conventional medicine refusing to explore other options than drug therapies is no reason for smoking to still be branded a lethal habit, and with enough people waking up to this fact, perhaps medicine will be forced to make breakthroughs. With smoking taking the blame for a range of illnesses, scientists simply have to pretend they are working on the cure, or produce more and more harmful and typically useless drugs, and just let smokers take the blame for the continued rates of cancers.

One area that deserves exploration into the onset of disease is that of genetics. There is a growing body of evidence to support this although, of course, it is still important to bear in mind correlation does not mean causation, and it is particularly tricky on the issue of genetics. For example, this book has already shown how social class has a huge impact on health, and in genetics it is almost unavoidable that a parent is in the same class as their offspring. Another important issue is that parents and children tend to have the same lifestyle – diet, exercise, outlook on life etc., and this obviously can have a massive impact. So whilst the topic of genetics is an important one, it is also important to keep in mind that the links may often be pointing to other causes too.

In the 1990s there was a much publicised study conducted by researchers at Johns Hopkins University School of Medicine. The study was looking at cancers of the head and neck and whether the p53 gene had any bearing on the onset or development of the disease; the p53 is the gene in a previous subchapter regarding lung cancer. The p53 was studied specifically because it is regarded as the Guardian Angel gene – believed to protect against cells becoming cancerous. A report in the March 16th 1995 edition of *Washington Post* stated that the researchers studied tissue samples from 129 people with cancers of the head and neck. The samples were divided into three categories: smokers, smokers and drinkers, and total abstainers.

The results showed that of the smokers and drinkers category, about 58% of the tumours had p53 mutations, compared to 33% from the smokers category, and 17% from the abstainers category. What can we take from this? While the statistics *may suggest* smoking and drinking is more likely to damage the p53 gene, two things must be remembered: firstly, every group had many participants with no damage to the gene, proving that an intact p53 gene does not mean cancer cannot happen; and secondly, every sample in the study had cancer! So whilst 17% of the abstainers had p53 damage and the remaining 83% did not, 100% had cancer. Thus, there is no question that a damaged p53 gene or a perfect p53 gene appears to make no difference to cancer, but perhaps it also tells us that the p53 gene makes a difference in the onset and development of cancer unless there is a genetic predisposition to the disease, in which case it will not keep a person from getting cancer. A good way to test this theory would have been to find out, of the 129 samples, how many of them had cancer in the family.

Tokuhata conducted a study looking at lung cancer and genetics by comparing the first-degree relatives of 270 lung cancer patients and 270 matched controls. The findings were that lung cancer deaths among non-smoking first-degree relatives of the cancer patients were almost four times that of the relatives of the controls, whilst there was no excess of deaths among the spouses of the cancer victims. The study concluded that the increased risk of cancer was down to genetics rather than environment or lifestyle.[118]

Whilst not to do with smoking or lung cancer, a very interesting study was conducted by DeFaire in 1974 (cited in Eysenck and Eaves, 1980), in which 197 same-sexed twins were

---

[118] Cited by Eysenck and Eaves in Asthon, H; Stepney, R. (1982) *Smoking, Psychology and Pharmacology* Tavistock Publications (p 127)

studied. When one twin died of ischemic heart disease, the other twin was investigated. The results were that in identical twins 94% of the survivors also showed evidence of ischemic heart disease, compared to 74% in non-identical twins. Of course, both identical and non-identical twins are related and share the same genes, and these results show a high risk of ischemic heart disease between siblings, despite living apart – seemingly leaving genetics as the only solution.

Before leaving this chapter, there is one more piece of evidence to show a link between cancer and genes. Despite pancreatic cancer being one of the rarest forms of cancer, it seemed to run in the family of former USA President Jimmy Carter – his brother, father, and two sisters all had it, and his mother died from breast cancer which metastasized to her pancreas. Obviously, lifestyle, environment and other factors cannot be ruled out, but given their high social status and expected healthy living, it seems genes certainly played a huge role in this instance.

# Chapter 6: Passive Smoking

Without doubt the single biggest weapon in the anti-smoking campaign, and resulting in the massive attention on public health, is passive smoking, or environmental tobacco smoke (ETS). Given that being told smoking was harmful did not stop enough people smoking to satisfy the anti-smokers, we were told that smokers are damaging the health of other people too. This has obvious implications: people can defend their actions by saying it is their body, their right, and ultimately does not affect anyone else; but being told that, actually, smoking tobacco will harm, and possibly kill, those around that person means that suddenly smoking is not just an inconvenience to non-smokers, but a threat to their health. Initially most people did not pay much attention to the warnings and shrugged it off, but in recent years the ETS campaign has grown with alarming speed, to the point where some people now claim smokers should be prosecuted for attempted murder.

There are, naturally, scary figures to accompany the scare; how else would we be convinced? It does not matter in the least to those creating the figures – and the hype – that no such danger really exists – this is all for the bigger picture: demonising smoking, at any cost.

This book has explained how, given the amount of people who smoke, it appears smoking cannot be killing as many people as we are led to believe – this can be determined without looking at studies, mere population statistics tell this. The fact the studies do not prove what they set out to also speaks volumes. But, if second-hand smoke is killing as well, then there would hardly be anyone left in the world today; if 80% smoked, 100% would be exposed to the smoke, meaning that, if we believe the official line, 50% of those active smokers would be dead, plus however many people passive smoke is supposedly killing (it is hard to say, given the figures change with rapid regularity).

In the late 1990s, the official number of smoking-related deaths in America was between 450,000 and 500,000. Dr Bernard M. Wagner, editor of *Modern Pathology*, said "Are there 450,000 smoking-related deaths per year in America? Maybe…but no human beings are ever studied to find out." We will look at how the numbers are calculated further into the chapter, but suffice it to say that Wagner is right – the death toll is not compiled by studying any actual humans, and the numbers are by no means accurate. It is interesting to note that statistically there are higher cancer risks from eating mushrooms, wearing a bra, or keeping a pet bird than there are from ETS.

In his book *Science Without Sense*[119] Steven Milloy discusses junk science and how, despite having the longest life expectancy in recorded history, public health officials are making billions annually by showing risks to health everywhere. It is an enlightening read, and some excerpts are included here.

> there's something of a gold rush going on in public health today. Thanks to the general public's neuroses about health, some strategic fearmongering, and, of course, political considerations, public health has struck it rich – to the tune of billions of dollars in annual revenues. Who would have thought it possible? It's the irony of ironies. More than half of us can expect to live past 75 years of age. Yet there are more public health professionals finding more public health problems than ever before!

He raises a good point – how is it that we are living longer than we ever have before when it is apparently miraculous that we survive at all, given the omnipresent dangers surrounding us? Of course, there *are* dangers about, and more worryingly there are dangers that were not there before, as a result of new technology and chemicals, and we will not know the dangers of these for many years to come. But it is also true, as Milloy pointed out, that given the current life expectancy is higher than ever, it is nothing but money that is responsible for the ever-growing number of 'dangers' we are exposed to.

Milloy then goes on to show how officials collect their data to scare people and reap large financial rewards. It is especially poignant because what he says directly relates to the methodologies used by anti-smoking researchers:

> What we're talking about is the kind of risk assessment that's not confined by the restricting chains of real science. Risk assessment that knows no shame, that will stoop to any level to achieve its self- fulfilling prophecies. In other words – assess for success!...This guide has everything you need to

---

[119] http://www.junkscience.com/news/sws/sws-preface.html

know about how to create a risk that will electrify the public, launch you into the pantheon of public health and land those big fat research grants from the federal government.

This relates directly to passive smoking because he goes into detail on why it is important to pick the 'right risk' for analysis – that is, something entirely improvable. He offers a guide to creating fear and offering the public bogus information to further the career of the researcher:

> The very existence of your risk must be unprovable by conventional scientific methods. After all, if it was provable, somebody else (like a real scientist), would already have done the work and your risk assessment wouldn't be necessary. A risk may be unprovable either because it doesn't actually exist or because the risk is too small to evaluate with science. In either case, fortunately for you, it's technically impossible to disprove such a risk...Using an unprovable risk offers several advantages. First, you can never be proved wrong. This is very important. Of course, you can never be proved right either, but that's a small detail, one that really doesn't matter in the grand scheme of things. You just need to allege, not prove.
>
> Second, an unprovable risk allows you to make outrageous assumptions about your risk, including the threshold assumption that your risk exists at all.
>
> Some of the more famous unprovable cancer risks are dioxin, electromagnetic fields, hazardous waste sites, environmental tobacco smoke, household radon, chlorinated drinking water and pesticide residue in foods.
>
> Your risk should be one that lots of people, if not everyone, come in contact with or are "exposed" to on a regular basis. But it should be difficult to impossible to measure how much exposure there actually is. This allows you to make up how much exposure there is and how to measure it.

Milloy has nailed it perfectly. The issue of environmental tobacco smoke (ETS), or passive smoke, is one that is just ludicrous and impossible to prove. As if the data for active smoking was not flimsy enough, the 'evidence' for passive smoking is even more so.

To anyone questioning the results or logic, the issue serves to undermine the entire anti-smoking crusade. Sadly, though, the public rarely look at the studies, let alone question them. The typical process is that the results are featured in the media, the public read or hear of them, and then regurgitate them with passive acceptance. It is no wonder that researchers get away with such injustices, and with the financial rewards they reap it is no wonder they continue. If this hounding of tobacco was legitimate then the government would have no problem funding pro-smoking groups such as FORCES to get a well-rounded and objective view of the analysis, and the researchers would let the raw data of their results speak for themselves instead of throwing out controls or adjusting the results unnecessarily. The fact is, though, neither of these things happen, and that really speaks volumes. Somehow, the anti-smoking brigade has also managed to demonise the tobacco companies nowadays to such an extent that people view them as evil and consider anything they say to be lies. These people forget that the tobacco companies nowadays actually boast that their products are harmful, as doing so prevents lawsuits against them (more on this in chapter twelve), and simultaneous to hating Big Tobacco they believe the words of other companies, such as Monsanto, who sell dangerous products and not only deny a risk, but outright say their product is safe.

Milloy also makes very sharp critique of epidemiological studies. Or, rather, he criticises the way they are used nowadays:

> There are two basic types of epidemiology studies that you can perform – cohort and case-control. Avoid cohort studies. They involve following a specific group of people into the distant future. Although cohort studies are the better type of epidemiologic study, they can take 20 years or more to complete. You would have to put your ambitions on hold. By the time your results are in, the general public may have wised up and called a halt to the public health gold rush.
>
> On the other hand, case-control studies are preferred because they're fast. Instead of following a group of people into the future, you simply scrounge up a group you can look at in retrospect. It's like Monday morning quarterbacking, only better. At the end of this game, you can adjust the score almost any way you want.

'Adjusting the score' is certainly a trick the anti-smoking researchers are not averse to. Of course, if adjusting the results is necessary then the study failed to prove that a risk is present. It also means that the researchers are desperately trying to prove a risk exists, for reasons that serve to benefit them. One final quote from Milloy, this time on the language researchers use to convince the public:

> What does relative risk mean? Let's say you've studied the association between high fat diet and lung cancer. You've calculated a relative risk of 6. The correct interpretation of this relative risk is that the incidence of high fat diets in the study population was six times greater among those with persons with lung cancer than those without lung cancer. Now is that boring or what? This interpretation will take you nowhere fast.
>
> You need to reword and generalize this interpretation to give it some sex appeal. A risk assessor on the make would say something like "this study shows the risk of lung cancer is six times greater among persons with high fat diets." Notice how we've replaced "incidence" with "risk," two very different concepts and used the word "shows."
>
> "Incidence" means we merely observed the reported result in our study. "Incidence" does not imply, one way or the other, that a high fat diet is associated with lung cancer. By replacing "incidence" with "risk," however, we communicate that a high fat diet causes lung cancer. Our study didn't really say that, but don't worry. That's a small detail that the general public won't notice. Finally, use of the word "shows" implies the study proves the risk. In fact, with a single epidemiologic study, it's impossible to prove anything except the limited observations of that study.

Advertisers are more than aware of how a sentence is dressed up makes all the difference, and researchers are no stranger to it, either. Results of a study can have drastically different meanings to the public by the simple way they are worded. Whilst the real results would, perhaps, rouse the thoughts of someone, the dressed up report is intended to instil fear and convince them a real risk is present. It is this tactic, and the constant onslaught of 'new' evidence, that has garnered so much belief in the ETS story and caused millions of people around the world to believe that other people smoking will kill them.

Let us also look quickly at 'relative risk', as it is an important issue. Researchers find a relative risk associated with passive smoking and lung cancer to be at an average of 1.2, and the 2006 Surgeon General's Report states that second-hand smoke causes an increase of lung cancer and heart disease of 20-30% – a relative risk of 1.2-1.3. In science, a relative risk so low tends to have no impact and is typically regarded as a fluke, the result of bias or confounding variables, or simply that the product in question is nothing to worry about. The Editor of the *New England Journal of Medicine*, Marcia Angell, says: "as a general rule of thumb, we are looking for a relative risk of 3 or more before we accept a paper for publication" and Robert Temple, the director of Drug Evaluation for the FDA, says: "my basic rule is that if the relative risk isn't at least 3 or 4 forget it". So there it is: according to science and official members of scientific communities, the relative risk associated with second-hand smoke is not significant.

The statistics of cigarette consumption around the world have already been shown, and the United States of America has been used as an example of changing trends in smoking habits. Given that after World War II 85% of the adult American population was comprised of smokers and ex-smokers, nearly every single person in the country would have been exposed to second-hand smoke. If what we are told about smoking and passive smoking is true then we would expect to have seen a dramatic epidemic of lung cancer and premature death. Even if we accept the incubation theory we would have seen a lung cancer epidemic and a sharp decrease in the population in the 1960s or 1970s. However, not only did this not happen, the reverse happened and the population increased dramatically.

It is also important to realise that, despite what we may be led to believe, there is not an epidemic of lung cancer. In 1993, the American Cancer Society estimated that there were 153,000 deaths from lung cancer. At the same time, though, the United States has statistics showing that there were 2,140,000 deaths annually from all causes. If we compare the ACS figure of 153,000 with the figures in the *Statistical Abstract of the United States* for deaths from lung cancer, including deaths from "intrathoracic organs" i.e. oesophagus and the throat, the numbers are remarkably similar. It appears, therefore, that the ACS has exaggerated the number of lung cancer deaths by including cancers of the intrathoracic organs. However, even if we take the 153,000 as a given, that is a low figure considering there are over two million deaths from all causes annually, coupled with the number of smokers being in the millions and the sheer amount of people living in America we can see that lung cancer is relatively rare.

The Centers for Disease Control and Prevention (CDC) website informs us that, as a result of smoking, lung cancer has increased by 400% in women between 1960 and 1990. But is this really the case? As stated in the previous chapter, the rates of smoking by the 1960s had fallen drastically, and women were not new to smoking, thus even if the incubation theory is correct the rates of lung cancer would have increased for women at the same time as they did for men. It appears that, actually, the rise in lung cancer is a result of other factors including detection bias and increased diagnosis as a result of improved healthcare. Also, let us not forget that lung cancer is not the only type of cancer that has had a rise in occurrence. Julian Whitaker M.D. is a practitioner of alternative medicine and has his own newsletter on health and exercise, and in his October 1995 edition of his newsletter he stated:

> Since 1950, the incidence of all cancers in people between the ages of 50 and 60 years has increased by 44%, with even higher increases in some of the more deadly forms of cancer. Breast and colon cancer went up 60%, prostate up 100% and testicular cancer for men between the ages of 28 and 35 went up 300%. Lung cancer has gone up 262%, an increase that is obviously not related to cigarette smoking, because over the same period the number of people smoking cigarettes dropped from 50% to 25%.

Despite being a non-smoker who advocates refraining from smoking, he admits that the rise in lung cancer is unrelated to smoking as the rate of smoking dropped by 50% in the same time frame. The fact that other cancers have also risen serves to show that there is a general rise in cancer rates, not only lung cancer. This indicates that other factors are involved, such as increased diagnosis and lifestyle.

With regards to passive smoking, one of the most striking things is that there are no concrete figures. The statistics and figures are constantly changing, from a few hundred people dying annually, to multiple thousands dying annually. The fact is, if researchers or officials can see passive smoke is killing people they would have statistics to back that up. However, as Simon Clark, director of the smokers' lobby FOREST, said, there is no proof: "All we ever hear are estimates, calculations and statistics. Where is the hard evidence that people are dying of passive smoking?"[120]

Alas, the solid figures and evidence are not forthcoming because, simply put, they do not exist. In 2003, research published in the *British Medical Journal* appeared to conclude this, when the universities of California and New York analysed data from more than 35,000 people who had never smoked but lived with a spouse who did. They found no link between passive smoking and death from either lung cancer or heart disease.

In 2005 the president of FOREST, Lord Harris of High Cross, said:

> Proposals to ban smoking in all public places would be understandable if they were based on incontrovertible scientific evidence of harm to others.
>
> But this is very far from the truth. The truth is that the dozens of studies conducted around the world over the past 25 years fail spectacularly to yield any reliably stable, uniform or statistically significant link between lifetime exposure to environmental tobacco smoke and lung cancer in non-smokers.

He was right, too. Whilst there are many, many figures on passive smoking, none of them correlate with each other and they do not make a uniform figure to conclusively prove second-hand smoke kills. Without such information, how can we know passive smoking is a threat to health? The truth is, there is no way of saying, with the information we have, that passive smoke is a killer. Actually, surprisingly enough it turns out that even the officials themselves do not know where the numbers come from. There is an Internet News Group devoted to smoking, called alt.smokers. In the late 1990s one of the participants called the Office of Smoking or Health to find out how the government got to the estimate of

---

[120]http://www.guardian.co.uk/news/2004/nov/18/
thisweekssciencequestions.cancer

450,000 yearly smoking related deaths. The participant rang repeatedly, and different individuals within the government, only to find out that nobody knew the answer. One respondent told him the calculations might have come from a book entitled *Foundations of Modern Epidemiology* by David Lilienfeld, but they do not.[121]

Despite nobody knowing where the figures come from, we can see how the anti-smoking lobby generates false figures of 'smoking related' deaths. In April 1995 there was a letter written to the editor of the San Jose, Ca. *Mercury News* which informs us of the deception. Mary Ellen Haley, the author of the letter, explains that she lost a loved one to adenocarcinoma, and that seventeen days elapsed from the deceased's first visit to the doctor to the day of his death. Haley was provided with the information for the death certificate which she then took to the attending physician for completion. She then says that on the death certificate there was a line for the doctor to insert the immediate cause of death, and three lines for "due to". The doctor in question stated that the "due to" was cigarette smoking, which prompted Haley to question him and ask if he was sure the tumour was the result of smoking. The doctor replied he was not sure, but the ACS had issued guidelines to say that when a person dies of certain conditions and has smoked, the doctor is instructed to list the cause of death as smoking. In this instance, Haley persuaded the doctor to not put cigarette smoking as the cause of death, but this would be an exception and most people would not challenge the authority of the doctor. It is then obvious that the ACS guidelines produce a stream of figures that are attributable to smoking, even though it is not the case. Thus, we can see the official figures are actually falsified figures and in actuality mean nothing.

One way the numbers were calculated was using the 'garbage in, garbage out' (GIGO) method. GIGO is a phrase in the world of computer science which calls attention to the fact that computers will unquestionably process any input data and accordingly produce output data, irrespective of how ridiculous the input data was. At least one 'body count' of passive smoke deaths came as result of GIGO, using data from the 1993 EPA report which will be looked at later in this chapter. The fact of the matter is this: pumping data into a computer and then passing the resultant data off as solid fact is not science. A computer is unable to

---

[121] *In Defense of Smokers* www.lcolby.com

recognise confounding variables or the uncertainty of factors to health. Instead, it works on the basis that a certain percentage contracted an illness, therefore that percentage will remain constant over the entire population. For example, if an epidemiological study consisting of 10,000 participants found that eighty people who spend an hour in the sun contract skin cancer compared to forty people who spent half an hour in the sun, then the incidence is applied to the entire population. If we use America as an example, there are 300 million people making up the American population and that number is divided by the number of study participants, ten thousand. This is thirty thousand, which we multiply by fourty as that was the increased number of cancers for the group exposed to one hour of sun a day. The outcome is 120,000, and the news will then report that an hour in the sun a day kills that many people annually. Retired mathematician and scientist Rosalind Marimont wrote an insightful article into the 400,000 deaths per year figure.[122] In addition, we can see the breakdown of the age of deaths for people who died from a supposed smoking-related disease:[123]

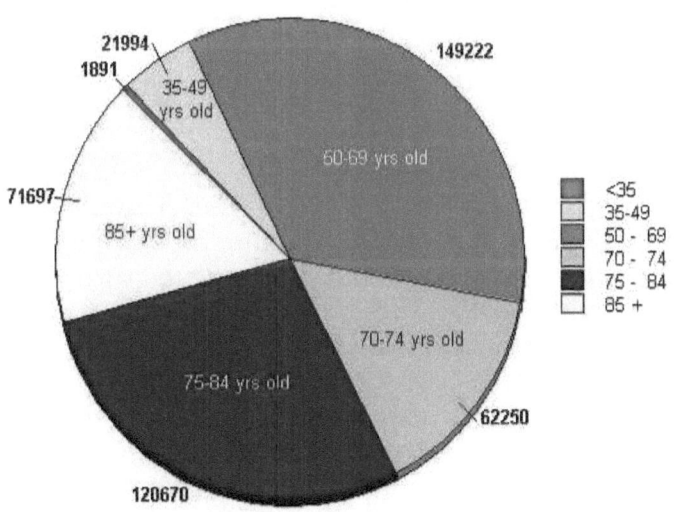

---

[122] http://www.forces.org/articles/files/sammec.htm

[123]http://www.geocities.com/madmaxmcgarrity/
SMOKERSANNUALDEATHS.htm

The chart clearly shows that the deceased are largely elderly, with over 120,000 being aged 75-84. Curiously, the largest group is aged 50-69, with almost 150,000 deceased. What is interesting is that the group has an age span of nineteen years, when the other groups range from four years to fourteen years. With the younger groups, such as 35-49, this is more understandable as cancer rates are low for people of that age. I suspect, however, that the 50-69 group is so large because the rates would have started to increase past the age of 60. Thus, the CDC can make it appear as though smoking is killing more people in middle-age than old age by merely increasing the category.

A large part of the success of the anti-smoking movement is that most people believe all health practitioners agree that smoking is a dangerous activity. However, this is not the case. The late Dr. Ken Denson of the Thame Thrombosis and Haemostasis Research Foundation said:

> I simply do not know where they conjure up their statistics. The statistics for passive smoking, in particular, would not be published or even considered in any other scientific discipline.

To those who do not know who Denson is, an excerpt from an essay by Joe Jackson is necessary:

> Dr Ken Denson, head of the Thame Thrombosis and Haemostasis Research Centre in Oxfordshire, who was a rare and inspiring objector to what he called the antismoking 'witch hunt'. Dr Denson had devoted ten years to researching smoking, and published several medical journal articles eloquently arguing that the evidence, if looked at impartially and in total, was equivocal. He had unearthed countless studies showing that changes in diet could offset any risks, that moderate smokers who exercised had less disease than nonsmokers, and so on, and simply wanted to know why such studies were ignored while anything appearing to show the slightest risk was trumpeted from the rooftops. In Dr Denson's view, doctors were failing smokers by preaching zero-tolerance instead of balance and moderation. He also suggested that we talk about 'smokers-related,' rather than 'smoking related'

diseases, since a majority of smokers have tended to have overall unhealthy lifestyles.[124]

It also transpires that studies show that diet affects lung cancer far more than passive smoke. In fact, the association between consumption of fruit and vegetables and rates of lung cancer is one of the strongest in epidemiology. There have been twenty-five published papers, and twenty-four of those show a clear statistical inverse relationship: the more fruits and vegetables consumed, the lower the incidence of lung cancer. The one remaining study found no association between diet and cancer. None of them provided negative results (that eating fruit and vegetables caused lung cancer). The results amongst all of them are very consistent in showing that those who eat less fruits and vegetables have a 50% increased risk of lung cancer.

There are also 156 published studies on cancers of the colon, breast, stomach, bladder, pancreas and ovaries, 128 of which show a protective effect of fruits and vegetables over contracting those cancers. Conversely, there are sixty-three studies of non-smoking women married to smoking males, only nine of which show a statistically significant positive association. Fifty-two of them found no link, and two show a negative association. In other words, studies on passive smoke causing lung cancer in women has only been successful 14% of the time, whilst studies showing a poor diet can increase the risk of lung cancer has been shown 96% of the time.

There is another important point to be raised here: it having been shown that diet has a huge impact on the onset of lung cancer indicates that the disease is not governed solely by the air quality entering the lungs. This simple point puts a big hole in the anti-smokers theory and their outcries that by eliminating smoking we can virtually eliminate lung cancer. This idea is nonsense, of course, given that there is no scientific proof that smoking has any link to cancer or disease of any kind, and the fact that with smoking rates having declined and reached a plateau, lung cancer rates have continued to rise, prompting many to realise that smoking was not to blame after all. With that key point shining through, it will not be too long before the crusaders look incredibly foolish – with

---

[124] Jackson, J. (2008) *http://joejackson.com/pdf/ 5smokingpdf_jj_smoke_lies.pdf* pg6

minimal amounts of passive smoke, fewer smokers than before, and lung cancer rates not dropping sharply.

Most people feel that the studies on smoking must be true and worthwhile otherwise they would not appear in medical journals. However, the journals are not the objective beacons they are considered to be. Their editors realised their publications could shape the opinion of the general public due to their relationship with a sensationalism-loving media. In fact, moral panics, a story or idea generated solely for hype with little to no basis in real life, have become a staple of society. As such, the media never turn down something that will cause hype and hysteria, and the medical journals love to deliver that. The following is a description of how the *Journal of the American Medical Association* (*JAMA)* released a story to the American media:

> the American Medical Association press office deluged 2,500 media outlets around the world with press packets, e-mails, faxes and, for broadcasters, tantalising chunks of ready-to-air film footage trumpeting the finds of the story.

This was published in a 1998 edition of the *New York Times,* at which time *JAMA's* editor was Dr. George Lundberg. Lundberg had just published a semi-completed study that attempted to show eating fish halved the risk of death by heart disease. The study was riddled with flaws and shortcomings, and when confronted about these Lungberg's response was "people are told that eating fish once a week is not a bad thing. What harm could it do?"[125] Well firstly, this is simple junk-science and a disservice to the public, given that the oceans are now so contaminated that seafood contains alarmingly high levels of mercury and other heavy metals that have the potential to damage humans. But what is most relevant about this comment, and study, is that it is the end-justifies-the-means approach, which has become synonymous with smoking – both active and passive.

Another good example of this approach can be found with Marc LaLonde. LaLonde is the former Canadian Minister of National Health and Welfare who argued that health messages should be "loud, clear and unequivocal" regardless of whether there was any solid scientific support for them. LaLonde felt that any

---

[125] Source: Snowdon, C *Velvet Glove, Iron Fist* www.velvetgloveironfist.com

study showing smoking was harmful should be released, regardless of how flawed it was, because it would convince people to stop smoking. It is amusing how people say anything that gets people to stop smoking is a good thing even if a study is wrong, because what they are saying is their opinion transcends the validity of science. Self-righteousness to the extreme.

One thing that is particularly damaging to the passive smoking theory is that the ACS has conducted a test on air quality, and discovered that ETS is up to 25,000 times safer than the Occupational Safety and Health Administration (OSHA) regulations for clean air. The American Cancer Society measured the air quality for second-hand smoke in several venues, and they tested by measuring nicotine (as nicotine is the only unique chemical since the chemicals in cigarettes are also found in the air and other places, thus testing for them would yield misleading results as the test would also pick up chemicals already present in the air). The results are shown in the following graph, ranging from 20-940 nanograms/cu.M. A nanogram is 10 (-9) of a gram, or 0.000000001 of a gram. The venues are, in order from left to right (lowest to highest): hospitals, restaurants without bars, restaurant with enclosed smoking area, restaurants with bar and dining area, restaurants with bar area, bowling alleys, bars/taverns, bar "Marlboro nights", and bingo halls.

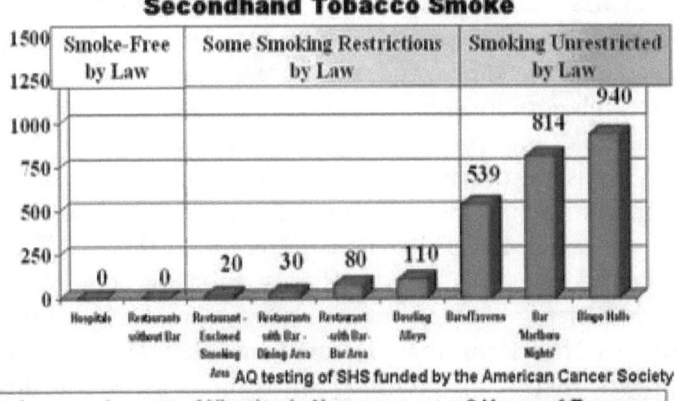

The

**Quality of Breathable Air for Western New York Workers: Comparison of Nicotine Particulate Levels in Secondhand Tobacco Smoke**

*AQ testing of SHS funded by the American Cancer Society*

■ Average Amount of Nicotine in Nanograms per 8 Hours of Exposure

OSHA has limits for air contaminants viewable in a table.[126] The OSHA safe exposure level to airborne nicotine for a full time job (forty hours per week, eight hours per day) is 0.5 mg/cu. M, as shown in the aforementioned table. In order to determine what the ACS air quality testing shows, the results must be compared with the OSHA permissible exposure limits (PEL). To do this, we divide the safe level (0.5 mg) by the ACS result of twenty nanograms, which is 0.00002 of a milligram. The result of 0.5/0.00002 is 25,000, thus meaning ETS is 25,000 times safer than OSHA regulations. The ACS have an upper reading of 940 nanograms, using the same calculation of 0.5 mg divided by 0.000940 we are left with 532. These results mean that ETS is safe by OSHA regulations, by anywhere between 532 and 25,000 times. In short: the ACS data indicates that tobacco smoke does not constitute a hazard to the health of those exposed to smoke, and a government ban on smoking in enclosed places is unjustified.

Further to the above, a letter from Greg Watchman, Acting Assistant Secretary of the OSHA, to Leroy J Pletten, PHD on July 8th 1997 read as follows:

> Field studies of environmental tobacco smoke indicate that under normal conditions, the components in tobacco smoke are diluted below existing Permissible Exposure Levels (PELS.) as referenced in the Air Contaminant Standard (29 CFR 1910.1000)...It would be very rare to find a workplace with so much smoking that any individual PEL would be exceeded.

What has recently become obvious to observers is that the groups pushing for the smoking bans are funded by pharmaceutical companies – the very same companies who are marketing a seemingly infinite supply of smoking-cessation items, such as gum, inhalators, and patches. The Robert Wood Johnson Foundation (RWJF) is an affiliate of the Johnson and Johnson Company, who happen to be the manufacturer of nicotine products to help people quit smoking. RWJF has issued a grant to the CDC, apparently to influence the CDC and officials to allow the tobacco Master Settlement Agreement funds to pay for smoking cessation products such as Nicoderm, manufactured by Johnson & Johnson. Thus, it appears that RWJF funding smoking bans is for their financial

---

[126]http://www.osha.gov/pls/oshaweb/owadisp.show_document?
p_table=STANDARDS&p_id=9992

benefits, as they believe that a ban will act as an incentive to many smokers to try and give up, therefore expanding their market and selling more products. Pharmaceutical companies, known as Big Pharma, spend an obscene amount of money on lobbying and have a huge amount of power as a result of their funds. Needless to say, this is not the place to expand on the lies and deception spewed by Big Pharma, but they have the power and money to convince people their products are worthwhile and necessary, despite being usually useless and harmful. We will look at passive smoking studies shortly, but the truth speaks for itself, and the truth is that the ACS has shown, positively, that second-hand smoke is not a health hazard. Furthermore, the official figures constantly change and are not backed-up by any evidence, and the official figures for "smoking related" deaths are entirely fabricated.

So, when did the passive smoking myth surface? The Environmental Protection Agency's (EPA) 1993 report[127] has been the basis for many of the accusations aimed at second-hand smoke, and also the basis for much of the legislation regarding it. In addition, nearly every subsequent study has been based on, or incorporated, the findings, premises and statistics from that report. Furthermore, the 'body-count' is nothing more than a computer generated estimate based on the statistical conclusions of the report in question – no wonder the figures keep changing, then, because they are literally created upon the statistics of a study.

Basing everything upon the EPA report would not be a problem if it were correct. As usual, it is *assumed* the report is correct and unquestionable, in other words, it is assumed the report is valid and objective well-obtained data. But, as we have come to expect from anything regarding smoking, this is untrue. It can always be tricky when a pro-smoker criticises anti-smoking figures, as people assume it is said to protect ones own interests, or to make a smoker feel better about smoking. However, no such accusations can be made when it is an anti-smoker criticising. This is exactly what happened when, in 1994, a Congressional inquiry[128] into the EPA and its methods concluded:

---

[127] http://www.tobacco.org/News/9807epawar.html

[128] http://www.pipes.org/Articles/Bliley.html

The process at every turn has been characterized by both scientific and procedural irregularities. Those irregularities include conflicts of interest by both Agency staff involved in the preparation of the risk assessment and members of the Science Advisory Board panel selected to provide a supposedly independent evaluation of the document.

What this means is that throughout the EPA report there had been "irregularities" including "conflicts of interest" – in layman's terms, there was significant bias and the results were the product of said bias, rendering them invalid. However, as a result of their methods, the EPA concluded that second-hand smoke was a Class A Carcinogen, meaning it is known, without doubt, to cause cancer in humans. This is very presumptuous given that even now, almost two decades after the report was written, nobody has managed to prove ETS as carcinogenic. The matter was taken to court and an anti-tobacco federal judge interviewed a range of scientists for four years, and subsequently portrayed the EPA report as an outright fraud and overturned that conclusion and the report itself. To quote the judge himself:[129]

> The Agency disregarded information and made findings based on selective information...deviated from its own risk assessment guidelines; failed to disclose important (opposing) findings and reasoning; and left significant questions without answers

and:

> Gathering all relevant information, researching and disseminating findings were subordinate to EPA's demonstrating ETS was a Group A carcinogen...In this case, EPA publicly committed to a conclusion before research had begun; adjusted established procedure and scientific norms to validate the Agency's public conclusion, and aggressively utilized the Act's authority to disseminate findings to establish a de facto regulatory scheme...and to influence public opinion...While so doing, [it] produced limited evidence, then claimed the weight of the Agency's research evidence demonstrated ETS causes cancer.

---

[129] http://www.forces.org/evidence/epafraud/files/osteen.htm

There we have it. The EPA resorted to the same tricks as Doll and the ACS in creating the results before doing their research, and then omitting any factors and controls that would have weakened their conclusion. Unfortunately this is nothing out of the ordinary in the world of anti-smoking but the truth does come out from time to time.

Judge Osteen was not the only objective reviewer of the report, and after analysing it the US Congressional Research Service said:

> The statistical evidence does not appear to support a conclusion that there are substantial health effects of passive smoking....Even at the greatest exposure levels....very few or even no deaths can be attributed to ETS.[130]

Anti-smokers may say that anyone can refute a report, and that such refutation means nothing. This may well be true, but there are two things to consider here: firstly, the reviewers are objectively analysing the report and have nothing to gain, financially or otherwise, by dismissing the report; and secondly, their analysis was not the only scathing review, in fact the report was criticised heavily by many different people and groups. Not every review is included here, but there are quite literally volumes of them available that go through the entire report and dissect it piece by piece.

A United States Department of Energy Report not only found serious flaws in the EPA's methodology but also demolished the underlying studies, and, extremely damaging to the report, quoted the EPA's prior critiques of the same studies. Confused? The EPA criticised studies as being statistically or methodologically flawed, and then decided to use them in their report as 'proof' that ETS was carcinogenic.[131] This just serves to show another example of deceit within the anti-smoking lobby. By 1993, there were thirty three studies on ETS, and over 80% of them showed no link between second-hand smoking and lung cancer. For their report, the EPA looked at thirty-one (discarding two reporting no statistically significant link between second-hand smoke and cancer) and came up with an estimate of 3,000 deaths annually from ETS.

---

[130] http://www.forces.org/evidence/files/crs11-95.htm

[131] *Choices In Risk Assessment* (1994) US DOE, Sundia Nat'l Labs

Of course, the EPA themselves did not believe this, as they had already heavily criticised the studies.

The Australian Supreme Court reached the same conclusion, saying: "The [study] results set out in tabular and statistical form did not support the claim of risk."[132]

The "important (opposing) findings" that Judge Osteen spoke of that the EPA "failed to disclose" were the results of one of the largest studies conducted up to that point, conducted by Brownson et al in 1992. The reason the EPA omitted these results was simply because if they had not then their premise would have been a no-starter. There are two reasons why Osteen's response had such little public influence: firstly, it had little publicity, which comes as no surprise as most things that contradict the general belief are largely ignored; and secondly, by the time it was released in 1998 there was simply too much at stake for too many people. By this time, it had become common knowledge that second-hand smoke kills, people had accepted it and as a result many careers were built on it and lots of money was collected, thus the conclusion of Osteen was overlooked.

There are two very important studies on ETS. The first was conducted by the World Health Organisation's (WHO) International Agency on Research and Cancer (IARC) and was meant to be the granddaddy of all passive smoke studies. The results were eagerly anticipated as definitive proof that ETS posed significant risk of increased chances of lung cancer, and no one would be able to refute this. The study ran for ten years and covered seven European countries, while the 1,008 female lung cancer patients to examine the sample size was double anything that had been conducted previously. Given the length and size of the study it is of no wonder it was considered the be-all and end-all study.

The results, however, were most certainly not what was wanted or expected. The study found no statistically significant risk for non-smokers living with or working with smokers, and, controversially, the only statistically significant link they found was that children with smoking parents were 22% less likely to develop lung cancer as adults, implying a protective effect of tobacco smoke.

Unsurprisingly, the WHO withheld the study until the *Telegraph* newspaper found it hidden within some other WHO

---

[132] *Federal Focus*, Vol. VIII, NO. 11, 1993

reports.[133] The WHO initially failed to make the findings public, and instead produced a summary of the results in an internal report. After the leaks reached the public, they issued a press release.[134] Despite lying in the title – *Passive Smoking Does Cause Lung Cancer - Do Not Let Them Fool You* – they did tell the truth in paragraph four:

> The study found that there was an estimated 16% increased risk of lung cancer among nonsmoking spouses of smokers. For workplace exposure the estimated increase in risk was 17%. However, due to small sample size, neither increased risk was statistically significant.

The WHO attempted to blame the results on having a small sample size, but we know they did not really feel this way because in the *Journal of the National Cancer Institute*, where the results were published, the researchers stated: "An important aspect of our study in relation to previous studies is its size, which allowed us to obtain risk estimates with good statistical precision"

The *Wall Street Journal* also covered the report on the 19th March 1998, and had this to say:

> For the past 15 years the antismoking lobby has pushed the view that secondhand cigarette smoke is a public health hazard. This was a shrewd tactic. For, having failed to persuade most committed smokers to save themselves, they could use proof that passive smoking harms wives, children and co-workers to make the case for criminalizing smoking.
>
> But the science fell off the campaign wagon two weeks ago when the definitive study on passive smoking, sponsored by the World Health Organization, reported no cancer risk at all. Don't bet that will change the crusaders' minds. The anti-smoking movement, after all, has slipped from a health crusade to a moral one.

---

[133] http://www.forces.org/articles/files/who1.htm

[134] http://www.who.int/inf-pr-1998/en/pr98-29.html

It is now obvious that antismoking activists have knowingly overstated the risks of secondhand smoke.

The findings of this study put the anti-smoking lobby on the back foot, and rightly so. As was to be expected, the usual personal attacks were made to those who condemned the report, with the *British Medical Association* calling the *Telegraph* journalists "mesmerised hacks".

The relative risk to a non-smoker with a smoking spouse of developing lung cancer was, in the findings, 1.16. Scientifically speaking, this is not statistically significant. When looking at relative risk we must also be aware of the odds of the number being a result of fluke. Statisticians have developed a few ways of working out if their number is generated by fluke, and the WHO chose the method known as the confidence interval which gives the range of results that the study might have reasonably produced if nothing more than chance was present. Unfortunately for the WHO, and all those hanging on the results, the study's confidence interval of 0.93-1.44 yielded a relative risk of 1, which is no extra risk. To encapsulate: the WHO's mammoth study, purported to have been the definitive study, found that, as the *Sunday Telegraph* stated, there is no threat of second-hand smoke causing cancer, and in fact it may even reduce the risk.

The second study of importance was commissioned by the American Cancer Society and funded by the Tobacco-Related Disease Research Program (TRDRP), entitled *Environmental Tobacco Smoke and Tobacco Related Mortality in a Prospective Study of Californians, 1960-98* in 2003, and it found the same results as the WHO study. The study, by researchers Enstrom and Kabat, focused on 35,561 Californians who had never smoked but who were married to smokers. They were followed for thirty-nine years by the ACS, from 1959 to 1998. It is, to date, the largest prospective passive smoking study. The tabular results showed, without room for doubt or speculation, that there was no lung cancer risk whatsoever and even showed a slightly lower risk than expected among the general never-smoke population.[135] The anti-smokers are, as usual, claiming that the study was funded by the tobacco industry, even though it was funded by the ACS and the anti-smoking extremists themselves,

---

[135] http://www.bmj.com/cgi/content/full/326/7398/1057

with money from proposition 99 (more detail on Proposition 99 later in the chapter).

Gian Turci, former CEO of FORCES International said of the study:

> This study is a God send, as it has cancelled years of propaganda, misinformation and frauds, and it gives breathing space to the forces of liberty and truth to regroup and fight back against white-coated fascism, corruption of the health institutions – and the fraud of the century.[136]

What particularly highlights the level of propaganda and deceit within the antismoking lobby, and indeed the medical industry itself, is that when almost all of the data was collected the funding bodies revoked their funding, leaving Enstrom and Kabat to find alternate money. However, because the research to that point indicated no risk with passive smoking, no medical communities or bodies wanted to be associated with it, forcing the researchers to ultimately accept a grant from the tobacco industry funded Center for Indoor Air Research. Of course, some people will use this as an excuse to knock the credibility of the study but what must be remembered is that the data was collected *before* any tobacco industry money entered the equation, which is why the ACS and TRDRP pulled out. An important point must be made here: many people accept the anti-smoking figures because they come from studies, not taking into account that not all studies are equal. In order for a study to take place, it must receive funding and, as the above highlights, organisations will usually only fund a study that will yield 'good' results – that is, acceptable results. Neither the pharmaceutical industry nor the medical community want to be associated with a study that deems smoking as harmless, beneficial or anything other than incredibly dangerous. The truth of the matter is that 'pro-smoking' studies, for want of a better term, are hard to find not because smoking is so harmful but because it is rare to find a funding body that will allow such results to be obtained.

Another study of interest, partially because of the attention it received, is Britain's meta-analysis which was conducted by the

---

[136] http://www.forces.org/evidence/evid/bmj_study_articles.htm

Scientific Committee On Tobacco and Health (SCOTH).[137] The SCOTH report was the government's own, so the results were not difficult to predict in advance. This was released a week after the WHO's study and was timed to be released at the same time as No Smoking Day. Sadly, but tellingly, the study was nothing new and was just yet another off the factory line of propaganda in the name of science, and it included no new science at all – rather it just reviewed existing studies on second-hand smoke.

One problem with it is that middle age is defined as being between thirty-five and sixty-nine years of age – which is high by any standards, given the UK life expectancy is seventy-four for men and seventy-nine for women. So we can see from this that they willingly used misleading numbers to produce the desired results. In addition to this, the SCOTH report ignored the fact that almost 40% of the 120,000 deaths attributed to smoking occur in both males and females who were above the life expectancy.

In the SCOTH report, in the Environmental Tobacco Smoke section, point 2.7, a reference is made to a report by the Australian National Health & Medical Research Council (NHMRC) from November 1997. This report was blocked from release by an Australian court because the NHMRC had failed in discharging its statutory duty of public consultation. In April 1997 Simon Chapman, of the working party on the report, stated that the calculations of risk to non-smokers who were exposed to second-hand smoke to non-smokers were so low that journalists "will be hard pressed to write anything other than 'Official: passive smoking cleared – no lung cancer'."[138]

Despite this being another method of propaganda, they still found insignificant relative risks. On page three, point three, they say:

> SCOTH therefore concludes that SHS causes heart disease and that the best estimate of increased relative risk of heart disease in non-smokers exposed to SHS remains at about 25%.

---

[137] http://www.advisorybodies.doh.gov.uk/scoth/PDFS/scothnov2004.pdf

[138] *Free Choice* May/June 1997

25% is a relative risk of 1.25. On page seven, the SCOTH report acknowledges that the IARC monograph found a relative risk of never smokers married to ever smokers of 1.24, another statistically insignificant find. Tellingly, though, they claim this indicates a causal relationship between second-hand smoke and lung cancer. The final conclusion of the SCOTH report was:

> The causal effect of exposure to SHS on risk of **lung cancer** has been confirmed by further original studies and by the authoritative review conducted by IARC. The pooled increased relative risk remains in good agreement with that estimated by Hackshaw, Law and Wald at 24%.
> [emphasis in original document]

Thus, SCOTH found that a review of all the evidence on SHS showed a statistically insignificant relative risk of 1.24. Given that they could not change the numbers, they relied on public ignorance to convince people that 1.24 is, in fact, indicative of a causal relationship.

Finally, the majority of scientists named in the SCOTH report are well known within the anti-smoking movement. It is therefore of no surprise that the results showed what they did.

One study of particular interest is one conducted by Professor Konrad Jamrozik. The study is often quoted by Action on Smoking and Health (ASH) as they consider it irrefutable proof that passive smoke causes disease. Before looking at the study, it is important to look at the man himself. According to the Imperial College London,[139] Jamrozik is:

> a physician with an international standing in the field of tobacco control. Over the past decade he has contributed to a number of Australian national and state government reports on the subject, and as a high profile public health advocate he is willing to take a stand in the media. Last year he tackled the Australian Prime Minister, John Howard, on Western Australian radio about inadequate funding for quit-smoking campaigns.

---

[139] http://www.imperial.ac.uk/P2405.htm

He is a man with a clear agenda. It should be an obvious point that researchers should be objective and diligent in their studies, and any researcher with a pre-defined ideology on their subject of interest is not fit for such research.

The study in question was entitled *Estimate of Deaths Attributable to Passive Smoking Among UK adults: Database Analysis*[140]. The first problem with this study is in the title: it is an *estimation* of deaths caused by passive smoke. This means two things: one, the result is fully dependent on all the studies being analysed being correct in their methodologies and results, a point which we know is not true; and secondly, that Jamrozik is already convinced passive smoke is responsible for a certain number of deaths.

Jamrozik was interviewed by *New Scientist*, and the article provides some exposing information:

> Jamrozik's mathematical analysis used an epidemiological model to combine several sets of data. Death figures came from the UK Office for National Statistics for 2002 and information on what proportion of the population are exposed to smoke at work and at home was provided by ASH.[141]

ASH is not the home of reliable information; their mission is to rid the world of smoking, and it is an aim they are most vocal about. The figures they provided Jamrozik with were guaranteed to be unreliable, if not entirely fabricated. As a matter of fact, ASH's figures stated that 11% of UK workers are exposed to passive smoking, yet *Smoking-Related Behaviour and Attitudes*, published by the Office of National Statistics, claimed 8%. Had Jamrozik used the latter figure, his deaths from passive smoke would have been 27% lower at 417 instead of 652.

The study setting was "National UK databases of causes of death, employment, structure of households, and prevalences of active and passive smoking", which shows us that Jamrozik merely looked at the causes of death and where people are exposed to smoke, and drew conclusions. As if this is not flawed enough, we also know, as explained before, how the smoking-related deaths are

---

[140] http://www.bmj.com/cgi/content/abstract/bmj.38370.496632.8Fv3

[141] http://www.newscientist.com/article/dn4998

calculated. From the outset, then, Jamrozik was using flawed figures.

The *BMJ* provides room for people to comment on a study, and a consultant statistician took the time to comment on this one:

> Whereas previous estimates of risk from passive smoking have been limited to nonsmokers, Jamrozik produces much higher estimates of deaths by including deaths in smokers... There are other technical problems with Jamrozik's analysis. He assumes that, because 85% of adults aged 20-64 work, 85% of deaths in adults of this age occur in workers, clearly incorrect in view of the well-known "healthy worker effect". He also assumes without any support that at home and at work exposure are independent, again leading to overestimation of the risk. Failure properly to take age into account is also a potential problem. Among adults of working age, is the average age of workers in the hospitality industry really the same as that of the whole population, as implicitly assumed?... Overall, the paper must be regarded as speculative and unscientific, adding nothing to the debate on passive smoking.

Furthermore, there is this to consider:

> The vast majority of these are people over the age of 65, people who would have lived through much smokier environments than exist today. Clearly, their lives will not have been shortened by much even if Jamrozik's numbers add up. As for the supposed risks to bar and restaurant workers, the most prominent justification for smoking bans these days, we should note that it amounts to 54 deaths per year out of a workforce of well over a million – a risk factor of 21,000-to-one.[142]

In addition to this, Jamrozik included a note in his study which said:

> the calculations in this paper were commissioned by SmokeFree London, a collaboration of 33 local borough

---

[142] http://www.precautionarytales.net/2005_02_27_archive.shtml

councils in London concerned with extension of smoke-free policies in that city.

Figures provided by ASH, calculations commissioned by a group whom Jamrozik admits want an "extension of smoke-free policies", categorising deaths of twenty-year-olds with sixty-four-year-olds, and the assumption that all previous passive smoking studies are fully correct is what this study is made from. It is evidently not a study, but political advocacy masquerading as science.

The expected outcome of the ACS, WHO and indeed the information lurking within the SCOTH Report would be the end of the hype about passive-smoking being a killer and infringing on the rights of non-smokers. The problem is, though, that anti-smoking has become a political crusade rather than a health one, and that complicates things no end.

The World Health Organisation claims that second-hand smoke causes between 35,000 and 62,000 deaths annually from heart disease in the United States. However, the WHO fail to mention an important editorial from the *New England Journal of Medicine*. John Bailar, head of University of Chicago Hospital health studies, who is no friend of smoking or the tobacco industry, stated there is no known link between second-hand smoke and heart disease,[143] and then cited the poor quality of study data and evident researcher bias. An entire chapter has been devoted to heart disease further on in this book, but that point is relevant here to highlight how the WHO are selectively omitting important findings.

Not content with blaming smoking for just cancer and heart disease, the WHO also claim that:

> Second-hand smoke also causes and aggravates asthma and other breathing problems, particularly in children. It is also an important cause of sudden infant death syndrome (SIDS).

But researchers from the Centers for Disease Control and Prevention examining data from the Third National Health and Nutrition Examination Survey reported in January's Archives of Paediatrics and Adolescent Medicine that there was no association between second-hand smoke and asthma among 5,400 children aged four to sixteen years of age. As for SIDS, it is not known what

---

[143] http://www.foxnews.com/story/0,2933,26109,00.html

its causes are. In fact, in June 2001, Wake Forest University researchers reported SIDS may be related to a genetic deficiency, citing new research as showing that the absence of a particular muscle enzyme allows fatty acid products to accumulate, producing a toxic effect causing heart arrhythmias and respiratory arrest.

There are also other theories of what causes SIDS. One is that babies who die from the syndrome may have brain abnormalities that prevent them from waking up when they do not breathe in enough oxygen during sleep, which suggests that an 'immaturity' of the central nervous system is a likely cause of SIDS.[144]

A 2002 study published in *Acta Neuropathologica*[145] found that inadequate nutrition left some babies without all their brain neurons, thus leaving them at risk of SIDS by not being able to develop appropriate heart and lung control, with the researchers stating:

> We hypothesized that infants without the full complement of neurons and neuropil (ARCn hypoplasia) are at risk for SIDS because they are unable to develop appropriate cardioventilatory control during this crucial developmental period.

Another study from *Acta Neuropathologica* found there is evidence that SIDS may be related to fire retardants in the mattress the baby sleeps on.[146] Dr Mercola wrote in his newsletter:

> The mechanism is a common, ordinarily harmless, household fungus (Scopulariopsis brevicaulis) and certain microorganisms, which consume the fire-retardant phosphorus, arsenic and antimony in the mattress plasticizer.
>
> When the microorganisms in your baby's mattress consume the fire-retardant and other chemicals, they emit

---

[144] http://articles.mercola.com/sites/articles/archive/2008/10/28/fans-lower-risk-of-sudden-baby-death.aspx

[145] http://www.ncbi.nlm.nih.gov/pubmed/12070659?dopt=Abstract

[146] http://www.ncbi.nlm.nih.gov/pubmed/7523575?dopt=Abstract

neurotoxic gases including phosphine, arsine and stibine. The gas generation starts when the mattress and bedding warm up, due to contact with the baby's body.[147]

These studies show two critical things: firstly, the cause of sudden infant death syndrome is not yet known, and secondly, the theories that exist with scientific evidence show it is more to do with biological developmental problems than anything else, least of all second-hand smoke entering the lungs.

True to character, the anti-smoking lobby has yet to announce just why it is that there was not a big rise in asthma or SIDS between the 1940s and 1970s when rates of smoking were not only considerably higher than now, but smoking was also allowed just about anywhere.

Another study of importance is a German report from 2002 that spanned twenty-seven years, during which thousands of flight attendants were followed and monitored for cancer. Unlike most other passive smoking studies, this one did not use questionnaires to obtain answers. Further, the validity of the study cannot be attacked for bias on the basis of funding since it was not financed by the tobacco industry. An excerpt from the study reads:

> We found a rather remarkably low SMR [standardized incidence ratio] for lung cancer among female cabin attendants and no increase for male cabin attendants, indicating that smoking and exposure to passive smoking may not play an important role in mortality in this group. Smoking during airplane flights was permitted in Germany until the mid-1990s, and smoking is still not banned on all charter flights. The risk of cardiovascular disease mortality for male and female air crew was surprisingly low (reaching statistical significance among women).

Not only did the study not find a link between ETS and cardiovascular disease or cancer, it appears the researchers were expecting to find one, as they said the risk of cardiovascular disease mortality for both men and women was "surprisingly low",[148] which adds validity to the findings.

---

[147] http://articles.mercola.com/sites/articles/archive/2008/10/28/fans-lower-risk-of-sudden-baby-death.aspx

[148] http://www.data-yard.net/39/cabin.pdf

Finally, we will look at a research article from Alan Gross, from the department of Biometry and Epidemiology, Medical University of South Carolina. The article is entitled *The Risk of Coronary Heart Disease in Non-Smokers Exposed to Environmental Tobacco Smoke* and says:

> This article addresses the controversial issue of whether non-smokers' exposure to environmental tobacco smoke (ETS) increases their risk of developing coronary heart disease (CHD). Glantz and Parmley purport to provide toxicological and epidemiologic evidence in support of their contention that non-smokers who are exposed to ETS are more likely to develop CHD than non-smokers who are not so exposed. The toxicological evidence provided by Glantz and Parmley has been challenged by Wu and by Gori, among others. Moreover, the epidemiologic data considered by Glantz and Parmley are equivocal at best and do not include data from the American Cancer Society's Cancer Prevention Studies (CPS-I) and (CPS-II) and the National Mortality Followback Survey which, when added to the original epidemiologic database considered by Glantz and Parmley, indicate no statistically significant association. Furthermore, most of the epidemiologic studies indicate a myriad of biases and confounders that have not been adequately adjusted. Many primary risk factors that were identified in the premier heart disease study, the Framingham Study (Kannel et al.), including but not limited to ethnicity, family history, dietary habits, age, serum cholesterol, exercise and alcohol use, were either totally ignored or not adequately considered in the epidemiologic studies. It seems foolhardy, then, to claim an association as do Glantz and Parmley. But perhaps a more egregious breach of science is to predict a number of CHD deaths in non-smokers caused by ETS. Unfortunately, that is what Wells purports to do. When one considers all the available evidence, the only reasonable conclusion that can be reached is that no association has been established between ETS exposure in non-smokers and an increased risk of CHD.

All in all, a truly objective analysis of the available data leads to the conclusion that ETS poses either minimal or no risk. The Dutch

Parliament had a thorough and open-minded debate on passive smoke in 2005 and decided against a ban and instead proposed better ventilation measures and more non-smoking areas by 2009. They evidently found the evidence unconvincing; perhaps other governments need to re-assess their decisions to have blanket bans.

## Passive Smoking: A Political Issue

It is not unreasonable, given the lack of evidence between second-hand smoke and disease, to question why such large figures are branded about as factual and why the anti-smoking lobby is not retracting its statements that passive smoke is a killer. The answer to all this is that the issue is no longer one of health – if it ever was to begin with – but one of political agendas. It is of massive consequence when the member of a group against smoking speaks out to inform people of the lies being told. Dr. Elizabeth M. Whelan is such a person. Whelan supports the smoking ban for "aesthetic" reasons of non-smokers no longer smelling of smoke when they frequent a bar or restaurant, but feels there is little to no evidence that second-hand smoke is a direct threat to health.

On the 31st July, 2000, the Coalition for a Smoke-Free City ran a full page ad in the *New York Times*, lobbying the City Council for a complete ban on smoking in all restaurants, nightclubs and bars. In an editorial that quotes the ad, Dr Whelan, president of the American Council on Science and Health[149] – a group which in no way likes smoking – accuses her own compatriots of "alarmism", "hyperbole" and all out lying about the effects of second-hand smoke in order to push their agenda. She had this to say:

> the headlines...are alarmist: 'Secondhand Smoke... causes lung cancer, heart disease, asthma and respiratory disease... [and a sub-head goes on to claim], 'The #1 Killer in the American Workplace is... Secondhand Smoke.'
>
> What we have here is...hyperbole about the likely effects of secondhand smoke...the main message from this ad is that workers (such as bartenders) exposed to secondhand smoke are at significant risk of lung cancer and heart disease. [But] the evidence linking ETS with chronic disease is much more speculative than that...simply put, the role of ETS in the development of chronic diseases like

---

[149] http://www.acsh.org/

cancer and heart disease is uncertain and controversial [and your assertions are] without scientific basis.

By exaggerating, the Coalition only serves to give ammunition to those who...maintain that health advocates, motivated by the "end justifies the means" philosophy, frequently play quick and dirty with the facts in an attempt to justify the interventions they want.[150]

What more can be said? Dr. Whelan has said it all, and she herself is no friend of smoking, which means she has nothing to gain on any level by defending it. Whelan has also admitted what has been mentioned in this chapter: there are no actual bodies counted to come up with the numbers of how many people ETS kills:

The estimates of ETS caused deaths are guesstimates at best...Theoretical numbers...Maybe there are no deaths due to ETS in the workplace.

Further to all of this, Dr. Whelan has said possibly the most sensible and grounded thing ever to leave the mouth of an anti-smoker:

[S]cience-wise and PR-wise, I think we'd accomplish more...if we stressed the known, proven effects of ETS and dropped the theoretical charges.

Never was a truer word spoken. If, indeed, the public were to be presented with reliable, consistent and scientifically proven figures then the whole passive smoke campaign would have a lot more credibility and support. Instead, all that the public receives is unfounded estimates. Worse still, the estimates keep changing. Despite this, the citizens of the relevant countries are expected to believe all the new and ever-changing figures, despite there being no supporting evidence coming. If, as Whelan advocates, the anti-smoking lobby presented the *actual* known effects of ETS, it would be much more credible. She defines the known effects as "Irritation of the eyes, nose and respiratory tract and aggravated pre-existing asthma. Surely that is enough to justify [bans]." To this, she received the following reply "Surely it isn't. Your opinion on sufficient reason doesn't count here. It's the opinions of the legislators and city councils that count, and irritation isn't enough for them... That's why it's a bad idea." And another reply saying that there is no point

---

in having epidemiological guesses: "If we won't let it influence public policy. It's downright stupid...when we want those facts to motivate action."

It is a liberal use of the word 'facts' given that, by their own data and admission, they are not facts. At the end of the day, that is irrelevant to them. The figures and 'facts' only exist to persuade the officials to pass the desired legislature. As the above quote points out, the actual truth is not scary enough or convincing enough to warrant a ban and so figures must be fabricated in order to get the desired result. This just serves to prove Whelan's case that the anti-smoking lobby is

> motivated by the ends justifies the means philosophy [and] frequently play quick and dirty with the facts in an attempt to justify the interventions they want.

Dr. Whelan is something of a hero figure now, bringing truth and justification to all the lies and false 'information' spewed out at any given moment by the anti-smoking lobby. Mayor Bloomberg of New York in 2002 said "it's literally true that something like a thousand people will not die each year that would have otherwise died". On the ASCH website, Whelan had the following response:

> We are delighted that bars, restaurants, and offices in New York City are soon to be smoke-free — although we do question the means (municipal legislation) used to achieve this end. But what we are not delighted with is hyperbole about the alleged health benefits of such a ban.
>
> Who exactly are these 1,000 New Yorkers whose deaths Mayor Bloomberg claims will be prevented by his legislation?
>
> If, as we suspect, he is referring to deaths caused by exposure to secondhand smoke in restaurants and bars, the estimate of 1,000 deaths prevented is patently absurd. Our best estimate of the number of deaths prevented is somewhere between zero and a hypothetical ten to fifteen. There is no evidence that any New Yorker — patron or employee — has ever died as a result of exposure to smoke in a bar or restaurant.

Before anyone gets too excited and says passive smoking causes cancer in a theoretical ten to fifteen people, Whelan says: "theoretically, [10 to 15] individuals with severe asthma could suffer an acute, fatal attack in a smoky bar" and "[t]here is no evidence that any New Yorkers – patrons or employees – has ever died as a result of exposure to smoke in a bar or restaurant."

Could it be any clearer? No. All that is conclusively known about ETS is that it is annoying to many non-smokers, and that it can aggravate existing asthma – not cause asthma, cancer, or heart disease. A lie told a thousand times is still a lie, no matter how many people decide to believe it in the end.

One of the ways the anti-smoking lobby has become so successful is their primary tactic – anytime someone defends smoking or refutes the idea of a ban, he or she is attacked. Not physically of course, but their credibility is attacked by accusing that person of being involved with, funded by, or otherwise linked to the tobacco industry. Even if the involvement is far in the past, or even if there is no link at all, the accusation is still there. This convinces the public that all scientists, researchers and objective people condemn smoking and advocate the ban, and only those linked to the tobacco industry are against it. This could not be further from the truth. The following example is from an article[151] published on Junk Science, hosted by Stephen Milloy. Milloy, who is 'junk science' commentator for Fox News, includes links to the actual correspondence between involved parties:

> Americans for Nonsmokers Rights has had the courtesy (unwitting) to acknowledge that politics is more important to its cause than science. How did ANR come to make this confession?
>
> It started with [an] article[152] authored by Michael Siegel of the Boston University School of Public Health and posted on the ANR web page.[153]
>
> In the article, Siegel advises anti-tobacco activists "Do not get into arguments with the industry about scientific evidence...Instead, the best approach is to expose

---

[151] http://www.junkscience.com/sep99/anradmit.htm

[152] http://www.junkscience.com/sep99/anrorig.htm

[153] http://www.no-smoke.org/

the tobacco industry ties of the so-called scientists making the arguments."

In enumerating scientists allegedly on the payroll of the tobacco industry, Siegel wrote "Robert Levy and Rosalind Marimont released a report[154] (issued by the CATO Institute) attacking the CDC and its estimate that smoking causes 400,000 deaths each year. All of these authors have strong connections to the tobacco industry... Robert Levy works for the Cato Institute, which receives financial support from the tobacco industry and Rosalind Marimont is with the National Smokers Alliance which also receives tobacco industry financial support. (Note: Americans for Nonsmokers' Rights can provide copies of tobacco industry documents which reveal the details of these authors' ties to the tobacco industry.)"

In response to Siegel's allegation, Robert Levy challenged Siegel to provide supporting documentation,[155] [quote from Levy: "Yes, I accept your offer to 'provide copies of tobacco industry documents which reveal the details of [my] ties to the tobacco industry.' I'm not aware of any such document(s) but, considering the legal exposure if your allegation is without foundation, I'm sure you'll be able to substantiate what you have written and broadly disseminated over the Internet."]

Siegel's response indicated he would correct any misstatements, but he didn't think he made any,[156] [saying: "I did not intend to make any personal allegations about your ties to the tobacco industry...The only statement that I made was that the Cato Institute has received funds from the tobacco industry. This was information that was provided to me (with what I believe is adequate documentation) by Americans for Nonsmokers' Rights. Nevertheless, I will not disseminate inaccurate information. Please let me know if it is not true that the Cato Institute

---

[154] http://www.cato.org/pubs/regulation/regv21n4/lies.pdf

[155] http://www.junkscience.com/sep99/anrad2.htm

[156] http://www.junkscience.com/sep99/anrad3.htm

has received funds from tobacco companies, because if that statement is not correct, I will have it corrected immediately."]

Levy responded by pointing to Siegel's statement "Americans for Nonsmokers' Rights can provide copies of tobacco industry documents which reveal the details of these authors' ties to the tobacco industry." Levy asked for a retraction.[157]

Siegel admitted the article was misleading the way it was written and indicated that he asked ANR to post a retraction and apology.[158]

Levy accepted Siegel's retraction and apology provided it was posted on the ANR web site.[159]

Rosalind Marimont also took exception[160] with Siegel's article ["Your article in ANR accusing me of scientific corruption, and being bought by the tobacco industry is totally without foundation. Please produce the articles proving my ties to the tobacco industry. You say "Ms. Marimont is with the National Smokers Alliance" I am a member, and so are millions of other Americans fighting for fairness to smokers. You are obviously trying to persuade your readers that I derived financial gain from this organization."] and he apologized.[161]

Everybody happy? Not quite.

ANR refused to post Siegel's retraction and apology stating, "After further discussion...[and] input from other [ANR] Board members, we have concluded that the possible 'clarification' that you and I discussed is simply not feasible... I realize that your views on the matter are heart-felt and sincere, and that mere removal of your name from

---

[157] http://www.junkscience.com/sep99/anrad4.htm

[158] http://www.junkscience.com/sep99/anrad5.htm

[159] http://www.junkscience.com/sep99/anrad6.htm

[160] http://www.junkscience.com/sep99/anrad7.htm

[161] http://www.junkscience.com/sep99/anrad8.htm

the paper, without more, will not be entirely satisfactory to you. But at this point **ANR must put its political credibility ahead of what you consider to be your scientific credibility.**" [Emphasis mine][162]

This article is a perfect and prime example of the way in which anti-smoking organisations target and attempt to demonise any person who defends smoking, irrespective of their careers in science or health, and irrespective of whether they have actually received funding from the tobacco industry. The article is incredibly valuable as it is not mere speculation or hearsay; it contains every email from both parties during the exchange of words, which show verbatim quotes of the whole conversation. It is in this way that it can be seen, conclusively and without doubt, the deceit of the anti-smoking lobby. The emphasised quote above, posted on the ANR website, shows, direct from the horse's mouth, that the anti-smoking movement is run by a political agenda, not one of science or health.

A lot of people ask the question 'instead of a ban, why not have ventilation?' The truth is, there is no longer any excuse to have anything less than fresh air in a building as modern air-cleaning systems are able to suck out stale air and recirculate fresh air, thus keeping the air fresh at all times. Some people believe that a room without smoke is a room with clean air, but this is not the case – air contains less visible pollutants, carbon dioxide, carbon monoxide, radon and, as shown in chapter two, chemical carcinogens. Good air cleaners are capable of making the air in a building cleaner than the air outside, which is polluted with exhaust fumes. Tobacco smoke particles have been measured at about one micron, good systems can remove everything down to .30 of a micron. In fact, tests have shown the air in a smoking venue with a good air-cleaning system to be cleaner than the air in a non-smoking venue without one.

Further to this, the smell of the smoke in any decent establishment is barely noticeable. This all goes back to when smoking was allowed on airplanes and air purifiers were used to keep the air fresh, as soon as smoking was prohibited and the air purifiers removed, the stewardesses and passengers started to get ill from stale air. *Consumer Reports* analysed air quality in airplanes and

---

[162] http://www.junkscience.com/sep99/anrad9.htm

found it less than ideal.[163] This is not good enough for the anti-smokers, though, and James Repace, an anti-smoking crusader in the USA, stated that it would take "tornado force winds" to clear second-hand smoke from a bar. This is an outright lie, given that standard air-cleaning systems are widely used in laboratories using toxic chemicals, and for hospital infectious disease wards.

There is ample proof that ventilation works perfectly well, but the real crunch point is that permitting smoking in ventilated areas means the anti-smokers will have failed in their objective to obtain a complete smoking ban. It also means that the pharmaceutical companies do not get the opportunity to sell products to over a billion prospective customers.

In 1999 the Mesa AZ council passed a ban on restaurant smoking and a local restaurant chain, in a demonstration project, installed an air-purifier (or, in the words of an anti-smoker "some of the so-called new ventilation technology"). The same activist said:

> The council was approached by the restaurants, saying come and check [it] out and see what you think. The council contacted one of the tobacco control coalition members who visited the test site and indicated that indeed he couldn't see or smell smoke...The council took that to be a green light and voted an amendment to the ordinance allowing smoking...with this ventilation...[164]

So the anti-smokers themselves admitted that the ventilation system worked – tobacco smoke could be neither smelt nor seen. However, this was not good:

> The coalition got word that [engineering consultant X of the Y company] was in town, making the rounds with council members, providing in-depth information about the new technology. The coalition contacted ANR asking who [X] was, [learned that he] had provided testimony against

[163] *Consumer Reports* August 1994, pp. 501-506

[164] List-serv from internal correspondence between anti-smoking organisations during a 2001 attempt to strengthen the NYC ban

the OSHA [regulations] and that his company had been contracted by Philip Morris.[165]

So there is the proof. The anti-smokers themselves admitted that the ventilation system worked – the system that was neither manufactured nor installed by a company with interests in tobacco. However, it was renounced as a con job purely by being guilty of association. The bottom line is the crusaders had unwittingly dropped themselves in it, and as a result everyone is able to see the true motivation behind the smoking bans. The start of the ETS lie can be seen as far back as 1975 when, at a WHO conference, former British Chief Medical Officer Sir George Godber concluded:

> It would be essential to foster an atmosphere where it was perceived that active smokers would injure those around them, especially their family and any infants or young children who would be exposed involuntarily to ETS.

## Who Are The Anti-Tobacco Crusaders?

To begin with, the anti-smoking movement was made up by scattered individuals of probably no more than twelve or so people. Most people will probably ask 'how did such a small group get so much influence?' The reason is because of the members amongst them, which include James Repace, a physicist; John Banzhaf, a lawyer; and Stanton Glantz, a mechanical engineer, all of whom were in positions where they could use their influence to effectively promote and find funding for the wider movement. These individuals personally hated smoking and wanted something to be done so they would no longer have to tolerate it. Through misinformation, lies, damnation and, in Repace's case, a job at the EPA, they have succeeded in ostracising smokers as outcasts and implementing a smoking ban in all enclosed areas. We will look at Glantz first.

Stanton Glantz

---

[165] List-serv from internal correspondence between anti-smoking organisations during a 2001 attempt to strengthen the NYC ban

Glantz is a well known figure and no stranger to deceit, extending the mantra 'all is fair in love and war' to include 'getting your own way'. Stanton Glantz was a mechanical engineer who became a professor of medicine at a famous university (University of California) without acquiring a doctorate of medicine. How? Simple: by utilising the anti-smoking shortcut, wide open for those more concerned with ideology, politics, and selfish attitudes than science. Glantz was also involved with countless animal studies – including dogs, cats, rabbits and lambs – where he attempted to show how dangerous smoking and passive smoking is. Unfortunately for him, it did not work, given that no animal study has ever proved successful in showing smoking causes lung cancer according to the 1997 Minnesota vs. Tobacco court case. Glantz himself has spoken on how he approaches research:

> that's the question that I have applied to my research relating to tobacco: If this comes out the way I think, will it make a difference [toward achieving the goal]. And if the answer is yes, then we do it, and if the answer is I don't know, then we don't bother. Okay? And that's the criteria.[166]

What Glantz is saying is that he is far from objective, or indeed scientific. Glantz is a self-described "lunatic" anti-smoker, and he is such a prominent figure within the lobby that his name can be found in almost every area of the anti-smoking war. Despite not being a medical doctor, he claims to be an "expert" on every smoking-related topic, including, but not limited to: health, entertainment (censorship of smoking in films etc.), economics and social policy. He is a professor at the University of California (UCSF) and has been able to turn his hatred of smoking into a multi-million dollar goldmine by insinuating himself into government agencies, including the EPA and by appearing as a government-paid witness for OSHA,[167] as well as securing tens of millions of dollars in research grants for the university.

Glantz began his activism in the late 1970s when he founded Americans for Non-Smokers Rights (ANR) whose central purpose was to demonise smokers as social outcasts and to lobby

---

[166] Written Transcript Of 3-Day Conference *Revolt Against Tobacco* L.A., 1992 p.14

[167] http://tobaccodocuments.org/tplp/512682339-2498.html?
zoom=750&ocr_position=above_foramatted&start_page=11

for legislation to legally make that true through smoking bans. In the 1980s, he lobbied for a tax hike on California smokers (proposition 99) with the stipulation that a portion of the revenue be earmarked for further political activism by organisations such as ANR. In other words, Glantz wanted increased taxes on tobacco products so that part of the increased revenue could be rewarded to ANR – which basically was Glantz and his friends. It worked, too, with his initial take from proposition 99 being almost $500,000, and later a further $4million.[168]

James Repace – anti-smoker and, at the time, head of the EPA's Indoor Air Division – hired Glantz, as well as other anti-smoking crusaders, to contribute to the Division's "Technicial Compendium" on second-hand smoke. Given that at the time there was little known, and almost nothing established, on the effects of ETS, the compendium was, according to the House Sub-committee who later reviewed it, nothing more than "an advocacy document" made to appear as though it were science.[169]

What happened next really shows how malicious Glantz is. Before the draft of the report, which was later questioned and then publicly disavowed by the EPA, had been subjected to internal or peer review, Glantz violated EPA policy by leaking it to the press. As a result, Glantz succeeded in showing the public scary headlines, getting his agenda off the ground and becoming a celebrity. It did not matter to Glantz that the report was trash, or that he was violating EPA policy, he just wanted to get his own way. When the EPA director publicly disapproved the Repace compendium, and stated that some of its science was "a figment of Stan Glantz's imagination" Glantz responded by claiming the leak was a "mistake".[170]

In 1994 Glantz co-authored a study to prove that restaurants do not lose money as a result of smoking bans. To this day the study is widely cited by advocates of the ban. However, the study is no more objective or scientific than any of Glantz's other work. When the study was challenged as fraudulent and full of

---

[168] *Policing P.C.* National Review, Aug. 28,1995

[169] Ibid

[170] Ibid

errors, with towns without bans being counted as having bans, and losses being reported as gains, he refused to release his raw data. As we all know, the results of a study should speak for themselves, and when a researcher refuses to release the raw data they are digging their own grave and proving that their studies are false and biased.

In 1989, using money from proposition 99, Glantz decided to investigate California legislators. It was, of course, nothing but a political witch-hunt, and when his initial grant ran out he received a further $600,000 grant from the National Cancer Institute to continue the investigation. The subsequent report, *Undermining Popular Government*, released in May 1995, spent much time and money grousing about the diversion of Proposition 99 money from "tobacco control education" (i.e. Glantz himself) to such frivolities as health care for indigent children. It then attempted to make the case that this diversion was because of tobacco industry influence – not only on legislators, but on the California Medical Association itself, whom he described as "sleazeballs".[171]

Glantz then went on to list every industry contribution made to every politician over the course of twenty years and insisted that "incorrect" voters had been bought. According to Glantz, virtually every legislator had, at some point since 1976, taken such money. But, by his own logic, Senator A had been corrupted by $1400, yet Senator B was unshaken by $30,000, and L.A. City Council members had been bought for a mere $500.[172] It is worth noting that in Glantz's mind any opposition to smoking bans is "pushing the tobacco industry's agenda" – forgetting conveniently that not opposing the ban is pushing the ANR agenda. Glantz suggests that legislators who oppose the ban should be publicly attacked:

> In each state one or two politicians seem to be taking the lead in pushing the industry's position (at least publicly). As soon as these politicians start floating trial balloons, they should be attacked publicly. If they can be bloodied, it could

[171] *The Transcript of the Referenced Congressional Hearings* a.k.a. *the Bliley Report* http://www.pipes.org/Articles/Bliley.html

[172] *S.F. Examiner, Sunday Mag.* 6/2/96 Calling For Blood

well scare the others off. Fear is a great motivator for politicians.[173]

As far back as 1986, there are records of Glantz's advising New York activists – including some pretty powerful ones – on how to lobby the City Council by methods of subtle blackmail and threatened attack.

Glantz, however, got directly into the act by testifying, and importing others to testify, at the hearings that led to the first serious modern bans on smokers in 1995. Apparently, with a foreknowledge of both the proposals and the proceedings, which is information not available to ordinary citizens, he and his allies were essentially able to orchestrate the proceedings.

Stanton Glantz did not slow down as time went on. In 2001 he advocated a bill to widen the existing smoking ban from 95% to 100% of all New York restaurants. In pursuance of this the City Council had created Section 17-513.2, a "Second-hand Smoke Air Quality Task Force". This had been created to determine whether or not ventilation could be the answer instead of bans. Apparently, though, clean air is not what ANR wants, and Glantz renamed the body "The Pro-Tobacco Industry Ventilation Task Force", in keeping with his view that anyone who opposes his view – that smoking bans are the only solution – must be a front for the tobacco industry. True to form, Glantz spread the word that "many experts in ventilation are on the industry payroll, often covertly." And that "restaurant owners, bar owners, unions who install ventilation" are also industry fronts. Glantz even questioned the integrity of the head of the city council Peter Vallone:

> Vallone has consistently refused to remove the task force. In addition, Vallone's office has refused to disclose (to Business Week) who is demanding this task force.

Apparently Glantz ignored, forgot, or overlooked the fact that it was Vallone who had introduced the proposed bans and worked hard to get them. The anti-smoking crusaders, though, seem to think they have the power and control:

> [Though] advocates have lobbied hard behind the scenes to get rid of the task force…Vallone, has absolutely refused to remove it…The health groups think they will be able to

---

[173] www.smokescreen.org

control the task force once it is established...They are
fooling themselves...If the task force stays...then it is crucial
that the NY advocates kill the bill.

And later: "I urge the advocates in New York to either fix the bill or
kill it."

So much for it being up to legislators to fix the bills,
apparently the crusaders have that pleasure, which just goes to show
how much influence they have. It is also interesting to note the use
of the phrase "behind the scenes" particularly on the issue of
ventilation, as this was not exposed to the public. This was
undoubtedly down to the fact that public opposition would have
meant them ending up exposing their true goal – not to obtain
smoke-free air, but to obtain a world without smoking. Or, at least,
as little smoking as possible and certainly not where crusaders
might ever want to be. In 1990, Glantz let slip that a significant
motivation of the whole anti-smoking movement was to line
pockets and stop people like him being inconvenienced by smoke:

> The main thing the science has done on the issue of ETS,
> in addition to help people like me pay the mortgage, is it has
> legitimised the concern that people don't like cigarette
> smoke. And that is a strong emotional force that needs to
> be harnessed and used. We're on a roll, and the bastards are
> on the run.

## Joe Cherner

Joe Cherner was the founder and president of Smoke Free Educational Services, Inc., an organisation exempt from tax yet whose
major activity is lobbying. Cherner was also the Policy Chair of The
Coalition for a Smoke-Free City, a coalition of 250 groups including
major health charities in the local area. It is also the same group
who, in 2001, requested a full smoking ban in all restaurants, bars
and nightclubs. Most of the member groups are funded through
state and federal grants i.e. taxpayers' money, and also from the
Master Settlement Agreement, which comes from smokers. Thus,
smokers are paying to persecute themselves.

Cherner claimed to "identify with Spider-Man", no doubt
because of him being involved in spin, a business in which he
became involved with in the early 1990s when he started a
"crusade" to get tobacco billboards removed from Shea Stadium.

Being a man of extreme wealth, Cherner was able to put forth plenty of money into the crusade, and he invested $250,000 to target ETS. According to The New York Times:

> Mr. Cherner [offered] last year to donate $25,000 to the charity of Mr. Dinkins's choice in exchange for an interview. His offer was rejected...By contrast, Mayor Edward I. Koch met with him after Mr. Cherner offered to donate $100,000 to charities in exchange for a meeting.[174]

As Dinkins would not hold a meeting with Cherner, he did the only thing the crusaders know how to do: tried to smear the name of Mr. Dinkins. Cherner launched a $50,000 radio campaign which served to accuse Dinkins of being beholden to "tobacco interests". No surprise there, Joe Cherner and Stanton Glantz seem to share the same philosophy that if people oppose their ideology, they are somehow involved with the tobacco industry.

As predictable as Cherner's response was with the radio campaign, what made this incidence that much worse is that he was well aware the reason the tobacco billboards could not be removed was because the city had signed a long-term contract for them. Breaking the contract would have resulted in the city's Corporation Council and the Park Commissioner being sued. In other words, Cherner was well aware that the Mayor of New York was unable to remove the billboards, and not for personal reasons, but because it went against his ideology he attacked the name of Dinkins to the press and the public, acting like a spoilt child not getting his own way.

As well as the above activities, Cherner was also involved with two websites: "SmokeFreeAir.org" and "smokescreen.org" (no ties with this book), both of which work to lobby the New York City council. Cherner solicited mail from his national membership to the council. Cherner was also active behind the scenes in working to defeat the nomination of Christine Quinn, the Democratic politician and speaker for the NYC Council, to the chairmanship of the Health Committee. I have included messages that appeared on his site:

> The NYC Council will choose a health chair shortly. One of the candidates being considered is Chris Quinn. She is not

---

[174] *New York Times* "Anti-Smoker Presses Shea Billboard" 26th April 1993

in favor of smoke-free air and, in fact, she smokes!...What kind of message would the council be sending if it appoints Quinn as health chair?

He then lists alternative candidates and solicits irate mail. Note how Cherner is only interested in candidates who not only do not smoke, but are in agreement with his ideology of smoke-free air, showing that smoking is the most important problem he can see with New York City.

His efforts against Christine Quinn did not end with that message; he also posted on his website a copy of a letter he sent to Don Distasio, the Executive Director of the American Cancer Society:

> Don,
> There are 18 members of the City Council who have come out in support of a safe, healthy, smokefree work environment for ALL New York City workers. Councilwoman Chris Quinn is NOT one of them...Why does ACS want to endorse Chris Quinn for Health Chair when there are so many supportive Council members...? [S]he would be terrible for tobacco control. Who is determining this ACS position?[175]

Again, this serves to show his primary concern, and seemingly it is above other issues such as healthcare, crime, and other important political issues. His use of language is also telling – "tobacco control" sounds very similar to "alcohol control" in the prohibition era, which is apparently exactly what Cherner wants – tobacco prohibition.

### John Banzhaf

John Banzhaf is a name unfamiliar to many, yet he is the founder of Action on Smoking and Health (ASH). In 1966 he argued to the FCC that the fairness doctrine meant that anti-smoking messages should be permitted free air time as a counter to tobacco adverts. When charities, including the likes of the ACS, showed no interest Banzhaf decided to found ASH instead.

According to Banzhaf.net, he:

---

[175] www.smokescreen.org 15th January 2002

helped drive cigarette commercials off the air, and started the nonsmokers' rights movement by first getting no-smoking sections – and then smoking bans – on airplanes and in many other public places

and:

helped ban cigarette advertising in several European countries, and to ban smoking outdoors, in homes and cars where foster children are present, to protect children involved in custody disputes, etc.

Evidently, Banzhaf is a man with a huge superiority complex and is a very intolerant individual. ASH bills itself as the "legal action arm of the anti-smoking community" and provides anti-smokers with legal help in everything from taking custody away from smoking parents to "suing the bastards." The ASH website encourages people to file complaints and inform them of smoking parents with an anonymous tip, with Banzhaf saying: "all you have to do is prove it's [SHS] a nuisance and it's an irritation." He compares these cases to suing over a neighbour's smelly cabbage: "you don't have to prove it's a health risk, you just have to say, 'I shouldn't have to live with this stink.'"[176]

Any other person would be tolerant and accept the fact that people are free to make their own choices, whether it be smoking or growing cabbages. Banzhaf, though, has the idea in his head that his wants are more important than those of others. He is also of the opinion that smoking should be banned outdoors: "I think restricting smoking outdoors is the next major step in the nonsmoker rights movement" and perhaps in homes too: "the law is clear that individuals maintain no legal or constitutional right to smoke, even in one's dwelling." Perhaps someone should remind him that a constitutional right is not needed for something to be permitted – there is no constitutional, or indeed legal, right to exercise or eat sandwiches, yet both are permitted and acceptable. Someone should perhaps offer the counter-argument to John Banzhaf that since no constitutional or legal writing exists to say those rights are not allowed, this instantly suggests that they are.

---

[176] http://ash.org/

ASH has a list of victories on its site, some of which include: helped convince Montgomery County, MD, to ban smoking in all restaurants and bars; persuaded several major restaurant chains to review their policies regarding smoking; and helped formulate the legal theories behind the government's suit against the tobacco industry. These are just a few of their 'victories', ASH actually takes credit for over a thousand municipal smokefree ordinances across America.

To highlight further the sort of man Banzhaf is, here are some excerpts from the ASH website:

> That's right. Dozens of tobacco class action law suits – brought on behalf of current smokers, former smokers, families of former smokers, nonsmokers, and other entities – are currently pending, and could result in awards of many hundreds of billions of dollars.

> ASH's Sue the Tobacco Companies Information – Act NOW Before It's Too Late! This page tells you how and why you should sue tobacco companies.

> Please note, however, that this information is available only to member-supporters of Action on Smoking and Health (ASH). To find out how you can become a member of ASH on line, and to obtain access to this and other valuable information for members as well as several special gifts, please click here to learn the many benefits of joining ASH on-line, over the Internet.

James Repace

James Repace is a physicist and one of the most prominent anti-smokers. In an interview with Philippe Boucher he stated:[177]

> In 1976, I suddenly realized that indoor smoking created air pollution levels far in excess of any outdoor air pollution I had ever experienced. With Al Lowrey (an NRL theoretical chemist) I developed mathematical models for the

---

[177] http://www.tobacco.org/resources/rendezvous/repace.html

prediction of ETS levels, and collected field data and performed experiments to validate the models.

And

> In 1979, I went to work for the US Environmental Protection Agency in Washington, in the national Air Policy Office as a science policy analyst. I quickly made indoor air pollution an EPA policy issue, became an EPA media spokesman for indoor air, and was soon invited all over the country to speak on this emerging issue, and later testified before the US congress. In 1985, Al and I published the world's first risk assessment of passive smoking and lung cancer, estimating 5000 US nonsmokers' deaths per year.

What is particularly noteworthy is that he is very careful to use the words "prediction" and "estimating". This means, of course, that he has *proved* nothing, but has calculated numbers that he wanted to use and then spread them as facts. According to his Curriculum Vitae he all but invented second-hand smoke.[178] The opening sentence is:

> Identified SHS as a major source of indoor air pollution, and the greatest source of population exposure to respirable particulate air pollution (RSP), and developed equations for its prediction, in a ground-breaking paper that attracted international scientific attention.

The second point says "estimated that 5,000 lung cancer deaths per year were caused in the U.S. due to passive smoking in a risk assessment." The word "estimated" has appeared again because he was unable to demonstrate any actual deaths. The real classic, though, appears at the end of page one:

> performed the first measurements of SHS-RSP and SHS-PAH carcinogen concentrations in the hospitality industry before and after a statewide smoking ban, demonstrating that SHS contributed 90% to 95% of the pollution levels,

---

[178] http://www.repace.com/Repace-CV.pdf

massively exceeding air pollution levels served on a major U.S. interstate highway during rush hour.

I call it classic because Repace expects the public to believe that second-hand smoke "massively exceeds" air pollution levels on a motorway during rush hour. In other words, a night in a smoky room contains higher levels of air pollution than driving behind countless vehicles. Such constructs of imaginations are commonplace in the anti-smoking movement, but a little common sense demolishes them. Evidently, it did not occur to Repace that this cannot be the case, as proven by the fact that being trapped in a garage with a car engine running *will* kill you in mere minutes, whereas one can spend their entire days in a tobacco-smoke filled room and suffer no harm except perhaps a sore throat.

Considering the 'scientific' advances he made to fabricate the SHS data, his CV shows no medical education or science in the health field. In fact the "education" section of his CV includes only physics qualifications.

Repace has made his career from anti-smoking, he was in fact responsible for the now famous 1993 EPA Report on SHS, and he is not slowing down. He is now a "secondhand smoke consultant", and the homepage on his website states that he performs lectures on passive smoking, courses on environmental smoke science and policy, research and analysis, monitoring of smoke infiltration in apartments and risk assessment of individuals or the population for lung cancer, heart disease or asthma. The latter is highly interesting, not least because he is making such predications based solely on SHS exposure or cotinine in body fluids – forgetting, apparently, that cotinine occurs in the body through eating foods containing nicotine.

For a man who claims to know more about SHS than just about anyone else in the world, it is quite worrying that he thinks it takes winds of 300 mph to clear a room of second-hand smoke.[179] In fact, on the "Secondhand Smoke Fact Sheet" on his website, he claims it is a fact that

---

[179] both quotes from hearing before Montgomery County, MD, Council on proposed smoke ban

smoke-free buildings are the only remedy. Secondhand smoke cannot be controlled by ventilation, air cleaning, or spatial separation of smokers from nonsmokers.[180]

The claim that tornado-force winds are required to clear a room of tobacco smoke comes from a very dubious report he wrote. To give an idea of just how widely-accepted this ridiculous claim is, I will quote Christopher Snowdon, author of *Velvet Glove Iron Fist:*[181]

> Despite being intuitively ridiculous, the tornado claim has been repeated around the world. In addition to appearing six times on Repace's own website, a quick Google search reveals that it is currently being reported as fact by, amongst many others, ASH, Unison, Cancer Research UK, Americans for Nonsmokers Rights, the Clean Air Coalition, Smokefree Ohio, Stop Smoking Manchester, Smokefree Europe, the World Health Organisation and GASP (although the last three groups have settled for a mere 'hurricane').

The report itself was published by the American Society of Heating, Refrigerating and Air-Conditioning Engineers (ASHRAE) in 2005. Despite ASHRAE not being perhaps the most prominent of organisations, it was no accident that they were the ones who received the unpublished report. ASHRAE are the company that issue ventilation guidelines to the construction industry, and so if Repace could convince them SHS is simply unsafe and cannot be controlled indoors then he was much closer to realising his dream of smoke-free buildings. This would be perfectly acceptable if the report was scientifically sound, yet it is far from it.

Repace made two statements of particular importance: firstly, that the annual U.S. death rate from ETS exposure in bars is fifteen per 100,000 exposed; and secondly, that in a non-smoking bar the desired rate of ventilation is eighteen air changes per hour. Both of these points deserve further development. Fifteen per 100,000 workers is 0.015%. Put another way, Repace has decided that 0.015% of people working in a smoky environment die from it,

---

[180] http://www.repace.com/factsheet.html

[181] http://www.velvetgloveironfist.com

meaning they may have died from anything from lung cancer to an acute asthma attack. The fact that it is an estimation and not based on actual deaths proves that none of the deaths have been demonstrated to be caused by second-hand smoke.

The second point, that the desired rate of ventilation in a *non-smoking* bar is eighteen changes per hour is an extrapolation of an ASHRAE guideline that states this is the requirement for a *smoking-permitted* bar. Evidently, Repace has been tricky right from the start, changing requirements and fabricating numbers to meet his needs. To give an indication of how high eighteen air changes actually is, ASHRAE recommend private homes have a mere 0.35.[182]

Knowing that the number eighteen is fraudulent is bad enough, but James Repace then multiplied it by 6,750 to show that a bar requires 121,000 air changes each and every hour, or thirty-three per second, to have air quality that is as 'good' as a non-smoking bar. He even went on to say that "even greater airflow rates would apply for air cleaning, which inefficiently removes secondhand smoke gases". The number 6,750 is the result of some staggering manipulation. It starts with Repace's estimation of fifteen deaths per 100,000 per annum, which he then increases ten-fold to 150 deaths per million. This latter figure is then multiplied by forty-five, supposed to represent the forty-five years one spends working, which produces 6,750. First and foremost, this is all based on his own estimation. Worse still, though, is that it works under the presupposition that all bar workers work for forty-five years in that job, thus neglecting to account for temporary jobs, part-time jobs, those who do bar work to support themselves through university and so forth.

Moreover, the 6,750 is an estimate of deaths per lifetime, not per year. However, had Repace stuck with deaths per 100,000 instead of per million, it would have yielded a result of 675. Obviously, this number is not nearly high enough to induce panic and fear in people and so a multiplication was necessary. To quote Snowdon once more:

> considering that he is multiplying it by the number of air changes per *hour*, it would be more reasonable to also use the estimated number of deaths per hour. This, however, is

---

[182] http://www.ieqcorp.com/ventilation.htm

a figure of just 0.017 and it would have forced him to
conclude that 0.3 air changes per hour would render a room
safe – the very opposite of a 'veritable tornado'

Despite the abundant evidence that exists to show Repace was
fabricating figures left, right and centre to prove his point, many
accept his result and repeat it. However, more revealing than any
counter-study could ever hope to be is a real-life example. Thankfully, one exists. In Las Vegas in 1997, the Bellagio hotel and casino
opened. Installed was an effective ventilation system, the type which
Repace assured was useless and could not remove second-hand
smoke. The casino permitted smoking throughout with the
exception of the high-stakes poker room, and it was ventilated
several times an hour (but not nearly 121,000 times) with pure
outdoor air. Air quality tests were conducted in 1999, two years
after opening, and in 2005, eight years after opening. Both tests
concluded that the air was as clean or cleaner than that of outside,
but never inferior. The second test is most interesting, because it
shows conclusively that the air remained consistently clean despite
years of smoking taking place. Respirable suspended particulates
(RSPs) were found at between twelve and fifty-eight micrograms
per cubic metre, which is barely measureable, and less than half of
the RSPs were comprised by tobacco smoke. The OSHA has a safe
limit of five-thousand micrograms,[183] and some unventilated bars
only have four-to-six-hundred, which is considerably higher than
the Bellagio, but still far lower than the safe limit. In fact, all
chemicals tested for, including nitrogen dioxide, nicotine and
carbon monoxide, all fell well within the safe limits. These tests
prove conclusively that high-quality ventilation is an effective
measure against a smoky bar.

It is interesting to note – though unsurprising – that Repace
received a grant from the Robert Wood Johnson Foundation
(RWJF), shareholders of Johnson & Johnson. J&J is perhaps the
largest, pharmaceutical company in the world and the makers of
Nicoderm:

In 2002, Repace received a Robert Wood Johnson
Foundation Innovators Combating Substance Abuse award

---

[183]http://www.ornl.gov/info/press_releases/get_press_release.cfm?
ReleaseNumber=mr20000203-00

for his ground-breaking work on the effects of secondhand smoke. Funds from the award helped make this study possible.[184]

The bigger picture reveals that Repace is not a man with scientific integrity, nor is he a man who uses rigorous scientific methods to test his hypothesis. Instead, he creates figures and conducts senseless mathematical equations to prove his point. This is all conducted under the veil of science and public health, but in reality it is no more than his wanting to ban smoking because he has a personal dislike to it.

2006 Surgeon General's Report

Before leaving this chapter, it is fitting to mention some of the findings of the 2006 Surgeon General's Report.[185] The Surgeon General himself said that "Second-hand smoke exposure can quickly irritate the lungs, or trigger an asthma attack". It appears that he did not actually read the 2006 Report, as these were the findings relating to asthma:

11. The evidence is suggestive but not sufficient to infer a causal relationship between secondhand smoke exposure and adult-onset asthma.

12. The evidence is suggestive but not sufficient to infer a causal relationship between secondhand smoke exposure and a worsening of asthma control.

The Report also mentions Chronic Obstructive Pulmonary Disease (COPD):

13. The evidence is suggestive but not sufficient to infer a causal relationship between secondhand smoke exposure and risk for chronic obstructive pulmonary disease.

14. The evidence is inadequate to infer the presence or absence of a causal relationship between secondhand smoke exposure and morbidity in persons with chronic obstructive pulmonary disease.

---

[184]http://www.rwjf.org/programareas/resources/product.jsp?id=21651&pid=1135&gsa=1

[185] http://www.surgeongeneral.gov/library/secondhandsmoke/report

In chapter one, 'Introduction, Summary and Conclusions', pages thirteen to sixteen, the Surgeon General gives a list of what second-hand smoke does not cause. That list is:

1. The evidence is inadequate to infer the presence of a causal relationship between maternal exposure to secondhand smoke during pregnancy and spontaneous abortion.

2. The evidence is inadequate to infer the presence of a causal relationship between exposure to secondhand smoke and neonatal mortality.

3. The evidence is not sufficient to infer a causal relationship between maternal exposure to secondhand smoke during pregnancy and preterm delivery.

4. The evidence is inadequate to infer the presence of a causal relationship between exposure to secondhand smoke and congenital malformations.

5. The evidence is inadequate to infer the presence of a causal relationship between exposure to secondhand smoke and cognitive functioning among children.

6. The evidence is inadequate to infer the presence of a causal relationship between exposure to secondhand smoke and behavioral problems among children.

7. The evidence is inadequate to infer the presence of a causal relationship between exposure to secondhand smoke and children's height/growth.

8. The evidence is not sufficient to infer a causal relationship between prenatal and postnatal exposure to secondhand smoke and childhood cancer.

9. The evidence is not sufficient to infer a causal relationship between prenatal and postnatal exposure to secondhand smoke and childhood leukemias.

10. The evidence is not sufficient to infer a causal relationship between prenatal and postnatal exposure to secondhand smoke and childhood lymphomas.

11. The evidence is not sufficient to infer a causal relationship between prenatal and postnatal exposure to secondhand smoke and childhood brain tumors.

12. The evidence is inadequate to infer the presence of a causal relationship between prenatal and postnatal exposure to secondhand smoke and other childhood cancer types.

13. The evidence is not sufficient to infer a causal relationship between parental smoking and the natural history of middle ear effusion.

14. The evidence is inadequate to infer the presence of a causal relationship between parental smoking and an increase in the risk of adenoidectomy or tonsillectomy among children.

15. The evidence is not sufficient to infer a causal relationship between secondhand smoke exposure from parental smoking and the onset of childhood asthma.

16. The evidence is inadequate to infer the presence of a causal relationship between parental smoking and the risk of immunoglobulin E-mediated allergy in their children.

17. The evidence is not sufficient to infer a causal relationship between secondhand smoke and breast cancer.

18. The evidence is not sufficient to infer a causal relationship between secondhand smoke exposure and a risk of nasal sinus cancer among nonsmokers.

19. The evidence is inadequate to infer the presence of a causal relationship between secondhand smoke exposure and a risk of nasopharyngeal carcinoma among nonsmokers.

20. The evidence is inadequate to infer the presence of a causal relationship between secondhand smoke exposure and the risk of cervical cancer among lifetime nonsmokers.

21. The evidence is not sufficient to infer a causal relationship between exposure to secondhand smoke and an increased risk of stroke.

22. Studies of secondhand smoke and subclinical vascular disease, particularly carotid arterial wall thickening, are not sufficient to infer a causal relationship between exposure to secondhand smoke and atherosclerosis.

23. The evidence is not sufficient to conclude that persons with nasal allergies or a history of respiratory illnesses are more susceptible to developing nasal irritation from secondhand smoke exposure.

24. The evidence is not sufficient to infer a causal relationship between secondhand smoke exposure and acute respiratory symptoms including cough, wheeze, chest tightness, and difficulty breathing among persons with asthma.

25. The evidence is not sufficient to infer a causal relationship between secondhand smoke exposure and acute respiratory symptoms including cough, wheeze, chest tightness, and difficulty breathing among healthy persons.

26. The evidence is not sufficient to infer a causal relationship between secondhand smoke exposure and chronic respiratory symptoms.

27. The evidence is not sufficient to infer a causal relationship between short-term secondhand smoke exposure and an acute decline in lung function in persons with asthma.

28. The evidence is inadequate to infer the presence of a causal relationship between short-term secondhand smoke exposure and an acute decline in lung function in healthy persons.

29. The evidence is inadequate to infer the presence of a causal relationship between chronic secondhand smoke exposure and an accelerated decline in lung function.

30. The evidence is not sufficient to infer a causal relationship between secondhand smoke exposure and adult-onset asthma.

31. The evidence is not sufficient to infer a causal relationship between secondhand smoke exposure and a worsening of asthma control.

32. The evidence is not sufficient to infer a causal relationship between secondhand smoke exposure and risk for chronic obstructive pulmonary disease (emphysema and chronic bronchitis).

33. The evidence is inadequate to infer the presence of a causal relationship between secondhand smoke exposure and morbidity in persons with chronic obstructive pulmonary disease.

Thus, even the Surgeon General Richard H. Carmona was forced to acknowledge that passive smoking is not a causative agent of the long list of ailments that the tobacco control movement would have us believe. However, Carmona was a staunch anti-smoker, claiming to Congress at the start of his time as Surgeon General that tobacco products should be banned.[186] One month after making his statements, the Surgeon General retired, admitting that "science gave way to politics".[187]

He presented the results to the public in a drastically different light, thus failing to accurately portray the findings. For example, the Report mentioned an increased risk of heart disease and lung cancer among non-smokers who are *chronically* exposed to *high-levels* of second-hand smoke, although the relative risk found was actually still 1.2-1.3. Carmona reported instead that *brief* exposure increases the risk, stating in the press release:[188]

> Even brief exposure to secondhand smoke has immediate adverse effects on the cardiovascular system and increases risk for heart disease and lung cancer.

And to the media:

> Breathing secondhand smoke for even a short time can have immediate adverse effects on the cardiovascular system, interfering with the normal functioning of the heart, blood, and vascular systems in ways that increase the risk of heart attack.[189]

Carmona opted to neglect mentioning that exercising also has an immediate adverse effect on the cardiovascular system, in that it increases blood pressure, which is associated with strokes and heart attacks. This does not, though, mean that exercise causes such problems. Indeed, if we looked only at short-term effects then we would refrain from doing anything, eating causes an immediate surge of blood-sugar levels, which is associated with diabetes. However, we know that this subsides shortly after and eating is not only healthy, but essential to life. This indicates that to determine health effects of second-hand smoke, one must not look just at the immediate effect, but rather the long-term effect. Moreover, Carmona has made statements that contradict everything medical science has taught us. After all, heart disease does not develop

---

[186] http://www.consumeraffairs.com/news04/2006/08/surgeon_general.html

[187] http://www.consumeraffairs.com/news04/2006/08/surgeon_general.html

[188] http://www.hhs.gov/news/press/2006pres/20060627.html

[189] http://www.surgeongeneral.gov/news/speeches/06272006a.html

almost instantly, neither does cancer, and indeed even the official line maintains that smokers develop such illnesses after decades of the habit. It is, therefore, an impossible and illogical statement that brief exposure can cause such illnesses.

## Chapter 7: Smoking and Emphysema

Smoking is an easy target for any illness related to the lungs and respiratory system. As such, listing it as a cause of emphysema is a somewhat obvious choice. Yet searching for studies proving as much yields nothing. It seems evidence is little more than an avoidable nuisance in the minds of the anti-smoking crusaders. According to the NHS website, emphysema is

> a serious lung condition that affects the small air sacs in the lungs, called alveoli. The alveoli are small 'balloon-like' structures that are located at the ends of your bronchial tubes. After air has been inhaled into your lungs, it travels through the bronchial tubes and into the alveoli. It is here that oxygen is passed into the blood and carbon dioxide passes out.

> Emphysema causes the walls of the alveoli to break down so that larger air spaces are formed. The effect is that the total surface area available for gas exchange is greatly reduced. This means that less oxygen gets into your blood and there is a reduced supply of oxygenated blood to the muscles and vital organs. Also, the waste gas, carbon dioxide, is unable to pass from the blood back into the alveoli where it can be exhaled and, as a result, there is a rise in the amount of this gas in your blood. [190]

Typically, symptoms of emphysema show once 30-50% of lung tissue has been lost. Even more so than cancer, emphysema is a disease of the elderly, which leads to the obvious assumption that it is the result of genes and simple old age rather than an external cause. What we are told, though, is that tobacco smoke destroys the alveoli in the lungs, leading to the onset of emphysema. The NHS website states that the more a person smokes, the more likely they are to develop the disease:

> For emphysema, prevention is the best form of cure. By far the biggest preventative measure is to give up smoking. The more you smoke, the more likely you are to develop bronchitis and emphysema.

---

[190]http://www.nhs.uk/Conditions/Emphysema/Pages/Introduction.aspx?url=Pages/What-is-it.aspx

So not only is smoking apparently a cause of emphysema, but it is the main cause. An interesting idea, given that at one point over half of the American and British populations were smokers, yet there has never been an epidemic of emphysema, nor has it ever been the biggest cause of concern.

The first thing to observe are the rates of emphysema – overall cancer rates have shown an increase with a decrease in smoking rates, and according to Cancer Research UK lung cancer is the leading cause of cancer death. Thus it seems that finally we will start to see a change in attitudes that accepts that lung cancer is often caused by something else, so we must also look at emphysema rates. According to Health First[191] it is the fifth leading cause of death in the western world, and rates are increasing. The fact that rates are increasing is a tell-tale sign right away, seeing as smoking rates have declined steadily for decades. Calling it the fifth leading cause of death is very misleading as, according to FOX news, the figures are lumped in with other lung conditions (apparently caused by smoking) such as chronic bronchitis, and the total death rate of all these illnesses per year in America is 120,000. Emphysema on its own in America has increased from 2.3 million in 1982 to 3.1 million in 2002. This is interesting, as in that twenty year period smoking has not increased, which means at best the emphysema rates should have reached a plateau.

The figures in the above paragraph should be an embarrassment to anyone claiming smoking causes emphysema. In 2007, the population of America was approximately 301,139,947 – over 301 million people. Currently, approximately 25% of the adult American population smoke yet only three million people suffer from emphysema, less than 1% of the total population, and the total death rate from lung disease – excluding lung cancer – is only 120,000. These numbers are extremely low from a relative perspective, and saying emphysema is the fifth leading cause of death in the western world is surely to combat the figures. By not mentioning figures and simply giving such a scary portrayal, followed by 'emphysema is caused by smoking', people believe smoking is the cause of an epidemic. However, what is not mentioned is that even the fifth leading cause of death does not claim that many lives, relatively speaking, and furthermore it is not only emphysema but other illnesses such as chronic bronchitis.

---

[191] http://www.healthfirst.net.au/content/view/1092/42/

As with cancer, it appears that smoking has been used as a scapegoat to hide the fact that it is not conclusively known what causes emphysema. What is particularly interesting is the history of the disease. The 1973 edition of *Diagnosis and Treatment* says that the cause is unknown but "many doctors" think "cigarette smoking" causes it. In other words, during the time when smoking rates had decreased because people succumbed to the belief it was harmful, there were some doctors who felt smoking also caused emphysema – no doubt because smoking involves the lungs. In 1973 the definition 'Chronic Obstructive Pulmonary Disease' (COPD) did not exist, yet it is now discussed widely in medical textbooks as though the disease had existed and been recognised forever. COPD is simply an umbrella term for people with emphysema, chronic bronchitis, or both. Predictably, the cause is put down to smoking.

In the 13th July 1994 edition of *Washington Post*, there was an obituary of Richard Joshua Reynolds III who died aged sixty. Reynolds was an heir to the founder of the R.J. Reynolds tobacco company, and as such he was a particularly easy target – and pin-up boy – of the smoking/emphysema link. The photograph accompanying the headline showed Reynolds III smoking a cigarette, and an obituary stated he died from emphysema.[192] However, the obituary stated that Reynolds III had given up smoking eight years previously and that there was a family history of emphysema with his father dying from it aged fifty-eight – almost the same age as Reynolds III. The obituary also stated that the doctor of the deceased was unable to state the "immediate cause" of death. The fact that Reynolds III had stopped smoking aged fifty-two is important, as information on emphysema tells us that giving up smoking is the best form of prevention – meaning, then, that it is unlikely that smoking caused the emphysema in Reynolds III.

Whilst in 1973 there was no known cause of emphysema, there has since been a discovery of a genetic link and cause. In an article in the online edition of *Grolier's Encyclopaedia*, Howard Buechner, M.D., explains that a significant number of the people with the disease lack a gene that controls the liver's production of a protein called alpha-1 antitrypsin (AAT), and it is this protein which controls or degrades as enzymes known as neutrophilelastase,

---

[192] http://www.flatrock.org.nz/topics/money_politics_law/jim_corbett.htm

produced by the white blood cells. When this enzyme is left unchecked, it destroys alveolar tissue.

In fact, a 2004 book entitled *1-antitrypsin deficiency 3: Clinical Manifestations and Natural History* states that the deficiency of A1AT causes emphysema or COPD in adult life of virtually every person with the condition. There is also the proteinase/antiproteinase hypothesis, which says that normally the locally synthesised proteinase inhibitors, especially the aforementioned AAT, permeate the lung tissue, thus preventing proteolytic enzymes from digesting structural proteins of the lungs. Accordingly, lung destruction results from either an excess of proteinase release in the lungs, a reduction in the antiproteinase defence within the lung, or both. This leads to the conclusion that emphysema is the product of an increase in proteinase release.

It also appears that there is no proof that there is any other cause of emphysema than genetics or individual biology; the aforementioned lack of a gene may just be one factor, there may also be other genetic factors at play. Curiously, unlike with cancer, studies are very short on emphysema. If one searches for causes of emphysema what typically surfaces is AAT deficiency and cigarette smoking. However, unlike the AAT deficiency reasoning there is very little evidence of a link between smoking and emphysema, just 'assumed' information. It is claimed that centriacinar emphysema is a result of heavy smoking, but again there appears to be little substance to the claim. Even when smoking is claimed to cause emphysema the authors make sure to specify 'heavy' smoking and over many decades, and that emphysema is most often not discovered until the sixth decade of life i.e. when one is elderly. This information, coupled with the relatively low rates of the disease, imply that even if smoking *does* cause emphysema it obviously affects a small minority of smokers. Oddly enough, the most common type of emphysema is said to be centriacinar – the one claimed to be caused by smoking. Yet there are apparently no studies linking the habit to the disease, and scientists are telling us genetic deficiency of AAT is a cause of emphysema. Clearly the facts and fiction are getting intertwined somewhere.

In the 1982 14th Edition of the Merck Manual, COPD is introduced as a combination of emphysema and chronic bronchitis – with some sufferers having one or the other, and others having both. The book tells us that cigarette smoking "presumably" plays a role in COPD. On page 630 the book mentions the AAT deficiency and says it is a "rare condition". However, the language is vague as to whether this means the gene deficiency is rare, or that AAT causing emphysema is rare. It appears the language is intentionally vague, as if AAT itself is rare it is still the cause of most emphysema cases, whereas if AAT rarely caused emphysema the book would have no problem whatsoever in highlighting that as this would then implicate smoking as the cause.

Things had changed again by 1992, at which point smoking was blamed for COPD. In the 16th edition of the Merck Manual (1992) we are told that emphysema is caused by destruction of lung tissue caused by an unchecked enzyme. This is AAT, and is proof of the genetic link to emphysema. However, the book then states that smoking lowers the body's defences to the enzyme, yet fails to point out evidence or a reference for this. Thus, what we are left with is the fact that emphysema is relatively rare. Furthermore, plenty of smokers do not get emphysema, and plenty of non-smokers do. On top of this is the fact that the rates of COPD are increasing, whilst the rates of smoking are decreasing, pointing out that smoking cannot be responsible for this. Given emphysema generally appears in people over the age of sixty, even if we take the view that there is a thirty year gap before the disease becomes known it still cannot be concluded that smoking is a *cause*, because smoking rates started dropping over thirty years ago, meaning that emphysema rates would not still be rising now. Whilst it is indeed true that we would only see emphysema in people typically aged over sixty-five, that leaves us with thirty million Americans yet still only three million cases of emphysema, or 10%.

It also needs to be said that emphysema is not necessarily as debilitating as the general public appears to believe. It is a medical diagnosis which recognises there is a problem with the lungs, but plenty of sufferers live normal, unaffected lives and die as a result of something else.

Finally, the evidence points to emphysema being a genetic disease, as it is caused by a gene deficiency resulting in AAT going unchecked and destroying lung tissue. Add to this the fact that the evidence that smoking causes emphysema all by itself is not only somewhat arguable but merely speculation and wishful thinking, it transpires that smoking is most probably not a cause of emphysema or COPD.

# Chapter 8: Smoking and Heart Disease

Apparently, various cancers, emphysema, lung disease and a war on second-hand smoke is not enough for anti-tobacco crusaders. Their agenda is to ban smoking, and to do this smoking must be linked to as many health problems as possible. Predictably, smoking is now considered a cause of heart disease.

There is, though, a serious lack of evidence. Studies looking at risk factors of heart attacks and strokes have been conducted since the 1950s, when government scientists started to carry out studies in Framingham, MA. Three risk factors were identified early on: smoking, high blood pressure and cholesterol. However, these are by no means the only risk factors and well known ones now include fatty food (and foods containing hydrogenated or partially hydrogenated fats), excessive alcohol consumption, and lack of exercise. Oestrogen pills have been linked to heart attacks in women;[193] male pattern baldness has been linked to heart attacks in men;[194] and even more recently researchers have discovered a link between heart attacks and surplus iron in the diet,[195] with claims that the iron oxidises cholesterol and deposits harmful plaque on artery walls.

The problem with risk factors is that the researchers decide which ones to assess, and which to include in the final report. Further, it cannot be overstated that correlation does not mean causation – after all, 100% of lung cancer victims inhale air, and 100% of heart disease victims eat food, but everyone knows we cannot link breathing to lung cancer and all food to heart disease. Moreover, how can researchers be sure that a particular risk factor was responsible for the heart attack? The only way to deduce a risk factor is by isolating it as the one variable to which anomalous results can be attributed. As such, risk factors are automatically and without fail biased by the researchers' opinions, as they choose

---

[193] Bishop, J. E. 24th Oct 1985 *Studies Conflict on Estrogen Tie to Heart Attack* Wall Street Journal

[194] Ruffenach, G. 24th Feb 1993 *Baldness in Males and Heart Disease may be Connected* Wall Street Journal

[195] *Base Metal: Heart-Attack Study Adds to the Cautions about Iron in the Diet* Wall Street Journal 8th Sept 1992

which to include, exclude, study, and, ultimately, whether to reveal their raw data or to alter it to match their hypothesis or premise.

A good example of this is how, despite many people dying during exercise, no studies or research have really been conducted to determine if exercise is a risk factor for heart attacks. For instance, Jim Fixx, an accomplished runner and author of books on jogging, died of a heart attack whilst jogging. Apparently, Fixx had a history of heart disease in his family with his father dying aged forty-two from a heart attack. Some followers of Fixx have suggested his exercise added extra years onto his life, even though he died in his fifties. If the exercise did add years to his life, it still goes to show that if you are predisposed by your genes then there is nothing you can do to really extend your life far beyond its genetic limits. Similarly, Congressman Goodloe Byron died whilst jogging on the C&O Canal, after being warned by his doctor that he had a weak heart and should not over-exercise. Despite this, exercise is still lauded as beneficial to one's life and positive to health. Of course, exercise *is* beneficial to health and is necessary to ensure high fitness levels, but the fact does remain that, in some instances, exercise can be dangerous.

No matter what factors are analysed, there will always be ones that have been neglected. For instance, not too long ago in recent history many physicians would have disputed the idea that stomach ulcers were caused by bacteria, yet it has now been proven this is the case. Similarly, who would believe bacteria can cause a heart attack? Yet a study conducted in 2003 shows this could be true. The study was published in the June 11th 2003 issue of *Circulation* and shows that Italian researchers have found another link between inflammation and heart disease. The protein Chlamydia pneumonia heat shock protein 60 (Cp-HSP60) promotes inflammation and immune responses. Lead author and assistant professor of cardiology at the Catholic University of Rome Marzio Biasucci M.D. said the protein appears to be a strong indicator of heart disease and the breakthrough may lead to new ways to identify people at risk for it. He said "Ninety-nine percent of patients with acute coronary syndrome tested positive for Cp-HSP60 in their blood". Acute coronary syndrome (ACS) characterises patients with angina typically caused by atherosclerotic plaque disease or heart attacks.

The study consisted of 219 patients who were admitted to a coronary care unit with acute coronary syndrome, forty patients with stable angina who were free of chest pain for two weeks or more and 100 healthy volunteers (the controls). The participants were matched for age, sex and risk factors. Blood samples were analysed from all subjects at baseline and samples were taken again from forty-one ACS patients an average of 350 days later. The results showed that 99% (217) of the ACS patients were positive for Cp-HSP60, compared to 20% of the stable angina patients and none of the controls. Thus, the protein was only present in the patients with heart problems. The researchers also tested for high sensitivity C-reactive protein (CRP), which is a marker of inflammation linked with heart disease, not long before the study was conducted. They discovered that elevated CRP was "found in 60% of acute coronary syndrome patients, in 25% of the stable angina patients and in 8% of the healthy controls". The test was 99% effective in finding Cp-HSP60 and 94% accurate in ruling out the presence of Cp-HSP60. This is a spectacular finding, and one that has many possible implications for both the disease and treatment, yet it appears to be widely overlooked.

There are numerous studies on causes and risk factors of heart disease, and it is common knowledge that diet has effects on the heart. At least one study in recent years has shown that a diet high in fruits and vegetables has a protective effect on the heart that remains even if a person smokes – in other words, healthy eating protects against heart disease and smoking will not change this. The study was conducted by Dr. Kaumudi J. Joshipura et al, of the Harvard University in Boston, Massachusetts, and consisted of 84,000 female healthcare workers aged thirty-four to fifty-nine and over 42,000 male healthcare workers aged forty to seventy-five. Joshipura had this to say:

> Our data support a protective effect of greater consumption of fruits and vegetables, in particular green leafy vegetables and vitamin C-rich fruits and vegetables, against risk for coronary heart disease.

The investigators reviewed data from two large studies examining factors affecting the health of middle-aged people of both sexes. The findings were published in the June 19th 2001 issue of the *Annals of Internal Medicine* and show that people who ate the most fruits and vegetables were older, had healthier lifestyles overall and smoked less – but the relationship between high fruit and vegetable intake and low risk of heart disease remained regardless of exercise or smoking habits. What this says is exactly what was demonstrated in chapter three: that people who do not smoke tend to look after themselves better. However, what these findings also show is that, regardless of smoking habits, diet is extremely important in preventing heart disease.

The study also found that a high intake of fruits and vegetables lowered the chances of heart attack in people with type 2 diabetes, which is a potential complication of the illness. It is known that fruits and vegetables contain myriad compounds that have been linked with improved health, such as fibre, potassium, foliate and antioxidants, which have all been shown to lower the risk of heart disease.

Another study that goes against the belief smoking causes heart disease is one the American Medical Association has published in its archives entitled *Traditional Risk Factors and Subclinical Disease Measures as Predictors of First Myocardial Infarction in Older Adults*[196] in which the researchers stated "glucose level and systolic blood pressure were associated with the incidence of myocardial infarction, but smoking and lipid measures were not". Predictably, the AMA is remaining extremely quiet on this finding, and the press coverage is non-existent.

Just as the WHO conducted the largest ever study on passive smoking only to find out there was no increased risk of lung cancer as a result of exposure, they also conducted the largest ever cardiological study – to find no link between heart attacks and smoking. The study, known as the Monica Study, was published in the *British Medical Journal* in 1999. It assessed twenty-one countries over ten years and found the incidence of heart disease dropping across Europe, Australia and North America. Puzzlingly, the researchers found no statistical connection between this reduction and changes in obesity, smoking, blood pressure or cholesterol levels. The organisers of the study said: "changing rates of coronary heart disease in different populations did not appear to relate at all well to the change in the standard risk factors".

The study found that obesity rose around the world, smoking rates decreased in men and women, blood pressure dropped almost everywhere, and cholesterol levels remained steady. The researchers found no correlation between these risk factors and the incidence of heart disease. This comes back to the point made

---

[196] http://www.ncbi.nlm.nih.gov/pubmed/10386510

earlier that not all risk factors are known, and a study selecting risk factors is instantly biased by the researchers decision; choosing only these four factors meant others such as bacteria, genetics, stress levels and diet were all omitted.

In the 1970s a study was conducted to see the effects of smoking cessation along with other known healthy behaviours. To give credit to the researchers, they avoided the self-selection problem that skews results of epidemiological studies and the participants were chosen at random. The study group was called the Multiple Risk Factor Intervention Trial (MRFIT) Research Group.

The study consisted of 12,866 'high risk' men, aged thirty-five to fifty-seven, who were randomly assigned to one of two groups. Group one was a special intervention (SI) program in which there was drug-care treatment for hypertension, counselling to help stop smoking, and dietary advice to lower blood cholesterol – this group will be known as the SI group. Group two, the control group, were left to their own devices regarding their lifestyle choices.

The MRFIT Research Group released its first report in 1982, with an average follow-up time of seven years. The results showed no statistically significant difference between the mortality in the SI group and the control group in spite of the SI group having adopted healthier lifestyles.[197]

In 1990 the MRFIT released another report of ten and a half years worth of research with the same two groups. In this report, the SI group had a statistically significant reduction in coronary heart disease, however this was attributed to reduction in hypertension rather than smoking, as M. O. Kjelsberg, in the journal *Circulation* in 1990 stated:

> Two factors appear to have contributed to this more favourable mortality trend for the SI Group: (1) a change in the diuretic protocol for SI men about 5 years after randomization, which involved replacement of [one blood pressure lowering drug with another]; and (2) a favourable effect of intervention on nonfatal cardiovascular events during the trial years. In addition, delay until the full impact of beneficial effects on mortality end points from smoking cessation and cholesterol lowering could have contributed.

---

[197] *Multiple risk factor intervention trial*, 1982 JAMA, 248, 1465-77

In other words, the initial drugs were having, at best, no effect or, at worst, were killing the participants. By switching the drugs the participants had lower rates of CHD. The study found no evidence that smoking had any effect on CHD. Interestingly, there were more deaths from ischemic heart disease in the SI group than the control group, with the SI group having ninety-six deaths compared to eighty-six in the control group, and the SI group also had sixty-six deaths from cancer of the respiratory and intrathoracic organs compared to fifty-five in the control group.[198]

The health establishment tried to explain away the discrepancies of the study, with one group of writers saying that the higher incidence of lung cancer in the SI group involved smokers or ex-smokers, and there were no primary lung cancer deaths among those who had never smoked.[199] What must have slipped their mind was the fact that all the participants were chosen because they were deemed to be at high risk – there were no 'never smokers' in the group.

Another study using the intervention method is worth mentioning. In 1982 Rose, Hamilton, Colvell and Shipley reported on a ten year follow-up study of middle aged smokers who were believed to be at high risk for cardio respiratory disease. The smokers were divided into two groups: a control group, where the participants were allowed to continue smoking, and a SI group who were encouraged to give up smoking. In the SI group, half of the 714 men quit smoking. However, the results still turned up negative. Of the 714 men in the SI group, 17.2% died during the study, as did 17.5% of the 731 men in the control group – a difference deemed insignificant. Similarly, there was no significant difference with lung cancer – with twenty-five cases in the control group and twenty-two cases in the SI group – although there was a statistically significant increase of "all other cancers" in the SI group than the control group.[200] This showed that smoking cessation does not affect the rate of cancer or heart disease.

---

[198] *Mortality rates after 10-15 years for participants in the Multiple Risk Factors Intervention Trial,* 1990, JAMA, 263, 1795-1801

[199] Ockene, et al., 1990 "*Cancer in the Multiple Risk Factor Intervention Trial*", Am J. Public Health, 80 (8).

[200] Eysenck, H.J. (1991) *Smoking, Personality and Stress* Springer-Verlag Press (p13)

The final study in this chapter is one conducted in 2003 and is widely used to claim smoking bans protect heart disease caused by second-hand smoke. In April of that year, some doctors in Helena, Mt, released a study on the results of a smoking ban in that community. Helena as a city only has a population of less than 26,000, with a catchment area of approximately 66,000, and it has one hospital, so we can instantly see a problem with the study: the small sample. The study showed that during the six month period after the smoking ban was imposed there was a 40% drop in hospital admissions for heart attacks and that once the ban was lifted the heart attack admissions went back to the 'normal' level. The study has been criticised by Jacob Sullum (a senior editor at *Reason* magazine), amongst others, for a few reasons: the small number of people involved, the limited time period, and that the doctors conducting the study were supporters of the ban, meaning bias was almost a certainty. During the ban, twenty-six residents of Helena were admitted to hospital for myocardial infarction as opposed to an average of forty during the same period for the five years prior to the ban. However, Sullum raised a critical point: it is possible to find several six month periods during those five years in which the number of heart attacks was as low as, or lower than, the average of twenty-six recorded during the ban. Another point, which was mentioned in only a limited number of newspapers and reports of the study, including the *Milwaukee Journal Sentinel* on April 6th 2003, is that Stanton Glantz adjusted the figures in the report before it was released for "seasonal variations". Considering that the six-month period was the same as the preceding years, there was no need for such an adjustment. The unadjusted figures were never released, and neither were the number of admissions for the control period (the six months before the ban came into effect). This is always a sign that the researchers have resorted to trickery to get the results they want; if the raw data is not released, the researchers have not obtained the results they desired. It makes me wonder why Glantz was the one to adjust the figures, too. In addition to the fact they did not need to be adjusted in the first place, one would think if adjustments were to be made then they would be made by the researchers or doctors of the hospital. Given Glantz's agenda, and confession that the anti-smoking crusade is a political one rather than a health one, it is of little doubt that the original figures were not nearly as low as twenty-six and were probably nearer forty, if not forty itself or even higher.

A further criticism was made by researcher Geoffrey Kabat, who admits to be no friend of smoking: "I am in favor of vigorous smoking bans and feel there is no justification for nonsmokers to have to breathe air polluted with tobacco smoke."[201] He wrote in the *British Medical Journal* that:

> First, the researchers only had information from hospital records on where a person lived. They did not interview the patients, so they had no information on whether their exposure to secondhand smoke changed as a result of the ban. They also did not present any information on whether smoking habits were affected by the ban. The fact that they had no information on exposure is a major deficiency.
>
> Second, the drop in heart attacks is based on very few cases: 4 per month on average during the ban compared to 7 per month before. Due to these small numbers the reported difference could easily be due to chance or to some uncontrolled factor. The number of heart attacks in the area outside Helena was even smaller. It should not be surprising that, given these small numbers, there are fluctuations of the magnitude seen in this study.
>
> Finally, the "immediate effect" and its magnitude really should make anyone stop and question the connection the authors are asserting. There are few interventions in public health that have such an immediate effect. Even if all active smokers in Helena had quit smoking for at least a year, one would not expect to see such a dramatic effect. No previous epidemiologic study or community smoking cessation program has ever shown that a reduction in smoking or exposure to secondhand smoke causes an immediate decline in heart disease incidence or mortality.[202]

A further critique on the *British Medical Journal* website is from a senior house officer (SHO) at Weston General Hospital in Weston Super Mare, Kofi O Ofuafor. Ofuafor had the following to say:

--------

[201] http://www.bmj.com/cgi/eletters/bmj.38055.715683.55v1#56035

[202] http://www.bmj.com/cgi/eletters/bmj.38055.715683.55v1#56035

The authors admit to not knowing the prevalence of smoking and consequently the extent of compliance in venues affected by the ban, this is crucial as demonstrated by Rigotti et al. They showed a lack of full compliance in their study, furthermore Rigotti and his co-workers noted no change in the frequency of smokers in their law restricting smoking study.

The authors similarly conceded to not knowing the incidence of secondhand smokers during the study group, an omission which could at least have resulted to the observed effect.

Given an incidence of thirty-three percent of never smoked at admission during the study period,the authors failed to give the incidence for similar cohort of patients in the period immediately before and after their study.

We believe the size and methodology of the study by Glantz et al as admitted by the authors were further weaknesses of the study.

It is also noteworthy, that the study failed to stratify the age group of patients admitted for myocardial infarction during the study period as this may have supported the effect of smoking ban at work place especially if the incidence reflected a pre-retirement age group who are more likely to benefit from the effects of such a law. The study data was drawn from billing records which may reflect a socioeconomic bias. [203]

The Helena study has been rebutted countless times, and offers no evidence that second-hand smoke affects heart health. Despite this, it is used as proof that smoking bans lower heart disease incidence.

At the tail-end of 2005, author Michael McFadden and retired pharmaceutical chemist David Kuneman issued an article and outline of the results of a study that would have greatly impacted the chances of smoking bans being implemented.[204] The study, however, was greeted with almost complete silence with the

---

[203] http://www.bmj.com/cgi/eletters/bmj.38055.715683.55v1#56129

[204] http://www.acsh.org/factsfears/newsID.990/news_detail.asp

media practically refusing to acknowledge its existence. Both the publication of the Helena study and the refusal to publish the contradictory study from McFadden/Kuneman highlights the political rot within the medical community, including respected medical journals, and it perfectly explains why anti-smoking studies are so prominent in a variety of medical journals while positive or neutral studies are ignored. A short excerpt from the press release goes a long way in describing this bias:

> Medical journals have come under criticism in recent years for being influenced by large pharmaceutical corporations, putatively publishing research that favors expensive and profitable drug interventions while selectively suppressing contrary research. While we have not researched that question, our experience with having valid but "politically undesirable" research rejected by three journals (which should have felt a particular sense of responsibility to publish it) makes accusations of politicized publishing decisions at journals seem more plausible to us than it once did. [205]

It is a sad fact that medical journals, so highly revered and considered the havens of truth and objectivity, have become so politically motivated and involved, opting to follow what is desired over honest scientific research and reporting.

After reviewing the evidence, it transpires that there is no solid evidence that smoking is linked to heart disease. Whilst there are studies that *attempt* to link the two, they quickly unravel with a little examination. There are an abundance of studies showing no link between smoking and heart disease, including ones that have tried to prove a link, such as the WHO's Monica study.

Despite this, the notion remains and there is now the latest in fear mongering based on this: smoking causes impotence. Studying impotence would be one of the hardest things to do in terms of singling out a causative factor, and the paper *Smoking and Reproductive Life,* available on the Tobacco Control Resource Centre, states that circulatory and vascular problems are the most common cause of impotence, and that smoking is closely associated with atherosclerosis (fatty deposits narrowing the arteries). Therefore, it

---

[205] http://www.acsh.org/factsfears/newsID.990/news_detail.asp

turns out that the idea smoking affects the reproductive system is just a new hoax born out of the idea that smoking causes heart disease. Some time ago, there was a televised live anti-smoking meeting. One of the points raised was that young people do not worry about lung cancer because it does not relate to them, being typically a disease of the elderly. In response to this, the discussion turned to asking what young people do worry about, with responses including impotence for men, acne for both genders, and wrinkles and being overweight for females. Subsequently, funding has been sought and found for studies that perpetrate a link between smoking and the aforementioned. Thus, the notion that smoking causes impotence is utterly without merit, and relies on the equally meritless idea that smoking causes heart disease.

# Chapter 9: Smoking and Asthma

Whilst it is probably premature to say that most people believe smoking, active or passive, causes asthma, it is not premature to say that most people feel it is a risk factor for it. Certainly, the anti-smoking crusade is trying incredibly hard to convince us all that asthma can be caused by tobacco smoke.

There is no solid proof that smoking can be linked to asthma, less still as a causative agent. There is, of course, an abundance of junk science masquerading as real science and it is bandied around so quickly, forcefully and often that many people succumb to the fallacy that it is real science. The real science, however, shows asthma is entirely unrelated to smoking, except the ongoing idea that passive smoke may trigger an asthma attack. It is probably true that passive smoke can trigger an asthma attack, however it must also be pointed out that such individuals who are intolerant to tobacco smoke will also be extremely sensitive to car fumes and indoor irritants such as dust. Thus, it is not that tobacco smoke is so harsh as to start an attack, but in sensitive individuals any irritant can cause one.

A study published in the July 8th 2000 edition of the *British Medical Journal*[206] found very interesting results which challenge the mantra that smoke causes asthma. The study was an intergenerational study over twenty years and the researchers found that whilst the rate of asthma had doubled between 1976 and 1996, the smoking rate during that period had halved. Furthermore, asthma and hay fever increased for both smokers and non-smokers but more so for non-smokers, and the steep rise in asthma was dramatically underscored by the fact that prescriptions for steroid inhalants for treatment of asthma rose more than six-fold between 1980 and 1990 alone. What is extremely relevant, and telling, is that this pattern is not occurring solely in the population sample of the study: asthma and allergy rates are increasing drastically among adults and children in all developed countries, but not in less-developed poorer countries. Perhaps the problem lies in the fact that nowadays people have a suppressed immune system as a result

---

[206] Upton M N et al (2000) *Intergenerational 20 year trends in the prevalence of asthma and hay fever in adults: the Midspan family study surveys of parents and offspring* BMJ

of vaccinations at birth, antibacterial soap and hand wash, and going out of one's way to avoid smoke. All these things may appear healthy, but in actuality by avoiding these things the immune system becomes weakened and the body suffers a reaction.

The USA illustrates the pattern perfectly: during a period where smoking and exposure to ETS has declined significantly, asthma rates in both children and adults has risen to an all-time high. Between 1980 and 1995 the number of people reporting asthma in the USA more than doubled, from 6.7 million to 13.7 million,[207] which is a 75% increase in the rate per 100,000 population.[208] In addition, there was a sharp increase in the early 1990s and since then the rate has continued to rise, with the Centers for Disease Control estimating the 1998 rate at 17.3 million, or a 150% increase since 1980.[209] This will come as a shock to those who believe smoking causes asthma, as between 1980 and 1995 the rate of adult smokers dropped from 33.2 million to 24.7 million, a drop of 25%.[210] In the late 1990s the overall smoking rate stayed constant at 25% of the adult population – a number far lower than the 1966 peak of 42.6%.

Whilst asthma rates have risen throughout the USA, there are regional differences which show an inverse relationship between asthma rates and smoking and environmental tobacco smoke can be seen by comparing extremes between States. For instance, for a number of years California has had the second lowest rate of smoking anywhere in the United States – in 1998 its adult smoking

---

[207] Centers for Disease Control and Prevention, MMWR 4/24/98, *Surveillance for Asthma--United States, 1960-1995.*

[208] Centers for Disease Control and Prevention, MMWR 12/4/98, *Forecasted State-Specific Estimates of Self-Reported Asthma Prevalence--United States, 1998.*

[209] Asthma Prevention Program of the National Center for Environmental Health, Centers for Disease Control and Prevention, *At-A-Glance* (1999).

[210] Centers for Disease Control and Prevention, TIPS, *Percentage of adults who were current, former or never smokers...National Health Interview Surveys, Selected Years--United States, 1965-1995.*

rate was 19.2%[211] – and it had the strictest smoking bans to be found anywhere in the States. However, California has the largest estimated asthma prevalence in the USA at 7.1% in 1998.[212] The same sources tell us that Utah has had, for many years, the lowest smoking rate in the USA at 14.2% in 1998, yet the estimated asthma prevalence was 6.7%. Kentucky, in comparison, has the highest smoking rate in the USA and has only a few restrictions on public smoking. In 1998 Kentucky had an adult smoking rate of 30.8%, and an estimated asthma rate of only 5.9%. Somehow, then, the states with the lowest smoking rates have the highest rates of asthma, and the places where smoking is more prevalent have lower rates of asthma.

The rates of childhood asthma are increasing not only in North America, but Europe as well. Dr Talal Nsouli, of the American College of Allergy, Asthma and Immunology, states that the number of children in the USA with asthma has doubled in 15 years, whilst the rate for those under five years old has increased by 160%.[213] There is, however, a major difference between the asthma epidemics in Europe and America. In the USA asthma appears to be afflicting inner-city children and some of the ethnic minorities; for example, blacks and Hispanics have higher rates than non-Hispanic whites.[214]

Furthermore, neither maternal smoking nor second-hand smoke exposure during pregnancy seems to account for the ethnic differences. A study of 9,276 mothers, conducted by Beckett et al, concluded that:

> The prevalence of asthma among children of Hispanic (mainly Puerto Rican) mothers with one or more children older than 9 mo. of age was 18.4%, for blacks it was 11.3%, and for non-Hispanic whites it was 7.4%...In addition,

---

[211] Centers for Disease Control and Prevention, *Prevalence of current cigarette smoking among adults, by state and sex--United States, Behavioral Risk Factor Surveillance System, 1998.*

[212] CDC, MMWR 12/4/98 *"Forecasted State-Specific Estimates...."*

[213] Kim, Eun-Kyung, *"First Lady Launches Asthma Program,"* Associated Press, 4th May 1999.

[214] Centers for Disease Control and Prevention, MMWR, 4/24/98, *Surveillance for Asthma--United States, 1960-1995. Asthma Surveillance Summary*

increased risk for asthma in these children was not associated with higher reporting of environmental tobacco smoke (ETS) exposure.[215]

As a matter of fact, since maternal smoking rates during pregnancy began to be compiled in 1989 Hispanic mothers have consistently had the lowest smoking rates during pregnancy, compared to Blacks and Whites, whilst Whites have had the highest.[216] The following table has the data for 1989 and 1993:

|  | 1989 | 1993 |
|---|---|---|
| Hispanic | 8.0 | 5.0 |
| Black | 17.1 | 12.7 |
| White | 20.4 | 16.8 |

The table shows clearly that the smoking rates dropped significantly for all three groups, yet the positions did not change – that is, Whites consistently had the highest rate of smoking, Hispanics the lowest, and Blacks in between. Maternal smoking continued to drop after 1993, with 1995 having an overall rate of 14.0 and 1996 being 13.6, a 31% decrease of 19.5 in 1989. These figures indicate that smoking during pregnancy does not cause asthma, and has nothing to do with the epidemic of childhood asthma that is currently being seen. Furthermore, if smoking during pregnancy does not cause asthma, then it is quite ridiculous that exposure to second-hand smoke does.

Asthma rates are rising not just in children, but in adults in the workplace. An expert writing a book review in *The New England Journal of Medicine*[217] stated:

---

[215] Beckett, W.S. et al (1996) *Asthma among Puerto Rican Hispanics: a multi-ethnic comparison study of risk factors* Am J Respir Crit Care Med

[216] National Center for Health Statistics, *Mothers who smoked cigarettes during pregnancy, according to mother's detailed race, Hispanic origin, educational attainment, and age: Selected States, 1989-93*

[217] Xaver Baur, M.D., Book Review of Asthma in the Workplace [Ed. by L. Bernstein, M Chan-Yeung, J Malo and D Bernstein, New York, Marcel Dekker, 1999], New England Journal of Medicine, 342:15, April 13, 2000.

We know of more than 250 substances that can cause occupational asthma, and the list is expanding. Occupational asthma not only represents a substantial proportion of all cases of asthma but also is one of the main occupational diseases. The unsolved scientific questions concerning the increasing incidence of occupational asthma in recent decades, the socioeconomic effects of the disease, and prevention are the current challenges.

These ideas are supported even further by hospital discharge figures and the Centers for Disease Control and Prevention (CDC). According to The National Asthma Campaign, American Academy of Allergy, Asthma and Immunology, and Jim Pirkle MD, PhD, CDC's Environmental Laboratory, asthma incidence in under fifteen-year-olds has increased from 5.8 per 10,000 in 1970 to 35.8 per 10,000 in 1997. During the same period, smoking rates dropped from 40% to 24% and according to the CDC, exposure of children to ETS decreased 75%. [218]

In recent decades, there has been a serious crackdown on smoking in the workplace, especially since the 1980s. A government survey[219] noted that by 1992 there were smoking restrictions on four-fifths of all indoor workers, and there have, of course, been more bans subsequently – there is now a blanket ban on all indoor smoking in Britain except one's own home.

Perhaps what makes the asthma puzzle more confusing is that asthma is not the only thing on the rise – allergies are too. The National Institutes of Health say that fifty million Americans, or 20%, suffer from allergies.[220] Some people think they are allergic to tobacco smoke, which is unsurprising given it is currently the scourge of the developed world and people think it can cause just about any given problem they care to mention. As usual though, it is unproven that tobacco smoke contains antigens that would cause

---

[218] http://banthebanwisconsin.wordpress.com/2008/06/29/ets-and-asthma/

[219] Samuelson, R.J. *Smoking Fictions* Washington Post, 2/25/98, p.A17.

[220] Goetz, T. *Don't Inhale: Hotel Air Quality Becomes an Issue With Clients* The Wall St. Journal, 6/18/99.

an allergic reaction;[221] there are several studies using sham smoke and tobacco smoke with subjects who claimed to be allergic to tobacco smoke,[222] but these studies found no significant difference in the subjects' reactions to the sham smoke and the moderate or heavy tobacco smoke. Common sense alone will tell people that it is not possible for second-hand smoke to be responsible for allergic reactions, given that smoking bans have been in effect for a number of years, and the rates of smoking have dropped significantly, whilst the rates of allergies have risen rapidly.

I stated earlier in this chapter that it was my belief that at least part of the rising rates of asthma was down to such a clean environment. There is now less exposure to pets and smoke than ever before, everything is now very sterile with an abundance of cleaning products and so forth, as well as pharmaceutical drugs being administered for every problem, and parents rushing themselves and their children to the doctor for antibiotics at the first sign of illness. As a result, our immune systems have very little chance to develop, and as such when faced with dust particles and so forth the body is unprepared. Dr Fernando Martinez, director of respiratory sciences at the University of Arizona, is just one of an ever-increasing number of experts who have adjusted their thinking of asthma and now think asthma is, at least in part, caused by an overly-clean environment:

> Just as you need to use your eyes to develop sight and your legs to develop the muscles to walk, your immune system develops through its experience. By legitimately protecting our kids from dangerous infections we may have kept parts of their immune systems from maturing.[223]

Recent estimates say that 40% of American children are given antibiotics for a month or more before their first birthday, and Dr Martinez believes this is part of the problem. Further to this, there

---

[221] O'Connor, G.T. et al 1989 *The role of allergy and non-specific airway hyper responsiveness in the pathogenesis of chronic obstructive pulmonary disease* American Review of Respiratory Disease

[222] Urch, B; Shepherd, R.J., Silverman, F. (1985) *Pulmonary Function Responses to Passive Smoking and the Influence of Suggestibility* Health & Welfare, Canada

[223] Shell, E.R; *Does Civilisation Cause Asthma?* Atlantic Monthly, May 2000

is evidence that smoke exposure reduces allergic sensitisation, as published on Medwire News:

> Parental smoking during childhood and personal cigarette smoking in teenage and early adult life lowers the risk for allergic sensitization in those with a family history of atopy, according to the results of a study from New Zealand.[224]

Writing in the *Journal of Allergy and Clinical Immunology*, Robert Hancox, from the University of Otago, Dunedin, and colleagues explain that "the findings are consistent with the hypothesis that the immune-suppressant effects of cigarette smoke protect against atopy."[225] (Atopy is an allergic hypersensitivity affecting areas of the body that are not in direct contact with the allergen.)

Hancox and colleagues investigated the effect of passive smoking in childhood, and active smoking in both adolescence and adulthood, on allergic sensitisation in 972 participants in the Dunedin Multidisciplinary Health and Development Study. The study was a prospective longitudinal population-based birth cohort followed-up to age thirty-two years. The researchers stated:

> We found that children who were exposed to parental smoking and those who took up cigarette smoking themselves had a lower incidence of atopy to a range of common inhaled allergens.
>
> These associations were found only in those with a parental history of asthma or hay fever.

Of course, this book is not about what causes asthma and how to prevent it so I will not spend any more time deliberating on the subject. However, it needed mentioning as it is yet another illness that has been blamed on tobacco smoke, despite the fact the figures do not support this in the least. In fact, if we took the statistics at face value, it could be argued smoking has a preventative effect on asthma. Whether this is true or not we cannot be certain, but it does follow logically from the hypothesis that asthma occurs as a consequence of an under stimulated immune system.

---

[224] http://www.medwire- news.md/48/72330/Respiratory/
Smoking_linked_to_reduced_allergic_sensitization_.html

[225] Ibid

# Chapter 10: Smoking and Low Birth Weight

It is a commonly held view that pregnant women should not smoke because smoking is a cause of low birth weight. Once again, though, this is based on statistics and the idea that correlation means causation. As has already been established, the majority of smokers are from the lower social classes and those groups of people tend to be unhealthy, largely as a result of eating food of poor nutritional value. It is also an established fact that poor nutrition can lead to underweight babies.

This is probably where the answer lies: it is no secret that the food the mother eats is what helps her baby to develop, and thus food is very important. If a mother eats nutritionally poor food, her baby will not develop as well as it should have or could have. As a result she gives birth to an underweight baby. Women from a low social class not only eat unhealthy food but also smoke cigarettes. She gets labelled as a smoker rather than an unhealthy eater and thus when smokers are studied statistically it appears that smokers have underweight babies. This is interpreted as smoking causing low birth weight. Thus emerges an apparent statistical link between smoking and low birth weight.

Correlation does not mean causation, and in that example smoking is no more a causal factor than, say, reading a magazine (statistically, of course, most pregnant women will read a magazine. That in no way means reading that magazine results in underweight children though). In other words, the notion that smoking will lead to an underweight baby is nothing more than another ailment to afflict the lower social classes, and nothing more than proof that that group of people are unhealthier than people from the higher classes. An important point I have referred to more than once is that after World War Two, the majority of Americans smoked, with the figure of current and former smokers being approximately 85%. What this means is that if smoking really did lead to low birth weight, a whole generation (or at least, a very significant part of it) would have been underweight at birth, and given the baby boom of that period there would have been a high number. Accordingly, this would have led to increased infant mortality, and a higher incidence of illness and disease later in life. Then, in turn, the next generation would have been healthier and heavier at birth. This did not happen, and the life expectancy for the 1950s and 1960s was higher than it was for the 1930s and 1940s. Once again, looking at the bigger picture serves as an arrow through the heart of the anti-smoking crusade. Of course, a simple theory will not suffice to win the war, so a closer look at the evidence is necessary.

The NHS paper on low birth weight[226] devotes a large section to smoking and its effects on birth weight. One of the first things it says is that

> Babies born to women who smoke weigh on average 200g less than babies born to non-smokers. The incidence of low birth weight is twice as high among smokers as non-smokers (Messecar, 2001)

The incidence of low birth weight being higher amongst smokers does not mean smoking is responsible for the issue, it could just be a signal highlighting that the problem occurs largely in the lower classes, and thus the problem lies there – such as with their diets and lifestyles. The paper, and above quote, reference the findings from Messecar's 2001 study. The paper does not give the luxury of providing the study itself, but it does give a table with select studies, with the following headings: number and type of studies included; setting; participants; and protocol. It turns out Messecar conducted five controlled studies, all including measurement of low birth weight in addition to smoking cessation rates. The 'setting' was public clinics and management organisations in the USA and Sweden; the 'participants' were 2,266 women, and finally the 'protocol' was:

> Counselling provided by trained counsellors, self-help manual and literature targeted for pregnant women. All studies measured smoking status by salivary or blood thiocyanate, cotinine validation or exhaled carbon monoxide

In other words, the researchers did not ask the participants how much they smoked, but they measured the amounts of carbon monoxide and cotinine in their body and then worked out the chance of low birth weight compared to how high the figures of the chemicals were. The problem here is that the levels may be there from another source; for example carbon monoxide may be there as a result of living in a built-up area with pollution, such as a town or city. That problem renders the results of the study dubious at best,

---

[226]http://www.nice.org.uk/niceMedia/documents/
low_birth_weight_evidence_briefing.pdf

and trash at worst. Furthermore, we are not told any other factors. For instance, we are ignorant to the diet of the participant, the lifestyle, stress levels, workload, genetic history etc., and all these things could well play a part. It is very premature and unprofessional to simply pick smoking as the causative factor without first assessing the others.

The paper then goes into social class, and inadvertently proves my point and defeats their own:

> Smoking cessation in pregnancy is highly differentiated by socio-economic status, with women of lower education, income and employment status far more likely to continue smoking than women from higher SES groups (Graham and Der, 1999). Smoking in pregnancy is four times more prevalent among women in households in social class V than those in social class I.

Social class V is the lower group, and group I higher. So what we have been told is that women from higher social status are more likely to stop smoking, whereas those from the lower groups are not. This reinforces the claim that those in higher classes have better health than people from a low social status. Furthermore, it validates that mothers who smoke having underweight babies does not prove that smoking is responsible for that, but other factors such as diet and lifestyle are the real causative agents.

In 2001 Wanda Hamilton wrote an article about the evidence regarding maternal smoking and problems, such as premature birth and low birth weight.[227] The results of two Annie E. Casey Foundation reports showed that between 1990 and 1998 the rates of premature birth, low birth weight and prenatal care were all rising, whilst the rates of smoking were decreasing. Somehow, all over America these results were used on the news to explain how smoking during pregnancy was a big risk factor and needed to be avoided. None of the newsreaders questioned the fact there was an inverse relationship between smoking and pregnancy complications. But that is just what the evidence shows: an *inverse* relationship: as smoking rates decline, pregnancy complications increase.

---

[227] http://www.forces.org/research/files/none.htm

Whilst on the topic of smoking and pregnancy, the final word should come from Dr Richard L. Naeye, a leading obstetrical researcher who studied more than 58,000 pregnancies:

> We recently found no significant association between maternal smoking and either stillbirths or neonatal deaths when information about the underlying disorders, obtained from placental examinations, was incorporated into the analyses. Similar analyses found no correlation between maternal smoking and preterm birth. The most frequent initiating causes of preterm birth, stillbirth, and neonatal death are acute chorioamnionitis, disorders that produce chronic low blood flow from the uterus to the placenta, and major congenital malformations. There is no credible evidence that cigarette smoking has a role in the genesis of any of these disorders.[228]

---

[228] Developmental and Behavioral Pediatrics *Cognitive and Behavioral Abnormalities in Children Whose Motherrs Smoked Cigarettes During Pregnancy (*p425) December 1992

# Chapter 11: The Truth About Nicotine

Nicotine is undoubtedly a very misunderstood substance. Some people say it is carcinogenic, some say it is unique to the tobacco plant, some say it is the reason why people smoke. In actual fact, none of these statements are true. Nicotine is not carcinogenic, besides it being in foods like tomatoes, a food which many experts believes protects against cancer, it is also in products such as Nicorette – if it were carcinogenic, such products should not have been approved. As stated in chapter two, nicotine is in no way unique to tobacco as it is present in a range of foods. As will now be shown, nicotine is not the reason people choose, or continue, to smoke.

Firstly, there is now a fair bit being said about 'freebase nicotine'. BUPA, a private healthcare organisation in the UK, states on its website that:

> Freebase nicotine is the term used to describe a potent form of nicotine that is rapidly absorbed by the lungs and brain, causing a faster "hit".

> Freebase nicotine is absorbed in a similar way to drugs such as crack cocaine. For this reason it is believed to be more addictive than normal nicotine.

And:

> According to new research from America, some cigarettes may be more addictive than others because they release more of a particularly potent form of nicotine, called freebase nicotine.[229]

James Pankow, of Oregon Health and Science University in Portland, is someone who believes freebase nicotine is the most dangerous additive in a cigarette. In fact it is his study that BUPA refers to above as the "new research." He states that nicotine occurs naturally in tobacco plants in two ways, either an acid or a base, and that the acidic form is more stable and more concentrated whilst the basic form is known as "freebase" nicotine, and is more volatile. Subsequently, when it is smoked it is absorbed quickly and then rapidly reaches the brain. Note how Pankow thinks freebase

---

[229]http://www.bupa.co.uk/health_information/html/health_news/
060803nicotine.html

nicotine is an additive, because he then says that he and his researchers found the most freebase nicotine was in American Spirit – a brand of cigarettes that have no additives or chemicals whatsoever. In fact, American Spirit are so intent on keeping smoking true to how the Red Indians use it that they only use 100% leaf, and no reconstituted sheet tobacco or stem. Apparently, though, American Spirit contains 35% freebase nicotine compared to 9.6% in Marlboro, a brand that contains ammonia.

Pankow's study was published in the July 25th 2003 edition of the American Cancer Society's journal *Chemical Research in Toxicology*. What is most striking about the report is how it is based on assumption. For example, Pankow states "scientists have shown that a drug becomes more addictive when it is delivered to the brain more rapidly" and he uses that finding to assert freebase nicotine is therefore highly addictive without actually quantifying the data or testing his claim.

Apparently these researchers and health authorities are taking full advantage of public ignorance of nicotine. Nicotine, in today's usage, refers to a variety of chemical compounds that are derivatives of a specific base chemical – freebase nicotine. Confusing the two is not a good idea, it is much the same as comparing sodium chloride (table salt) with sodium hydroxide (a drain cleaner that reacts with fat, hair and human skin to make them water soluble). In actuality, the nicotine found in tobacco is a mixture of two "salts" of nicotine: nicotine citrate and nicotine malate. The nicotine in gum and patches is typically nicotine sulphate. Finally, the most common form of nicotine found in nature is nicotinic acid (otherwise known as niacin, or vitamin B3).

True nicotine, however, is called "freebase nicotine" which, unlike its various derivatives, is a strong reducing agent. This means it has chemical properties like metallic sodium and potassium in that it oxidises rapidly when exposed to air and reacts chemically with water, breaking water down into its chemical elements: hydrogen and oxygen. All green plants contain nicotine and use this property to break apart water molecules during photosynthesis. The specific forms of nicotine used during photosynthesis are nicotine adenine dinucleotide (NAD) and nicotine adenine dinucleotide phosphate

(NADP). Furthermore, all living cells use NAD and NADP to release energy from sugar molecules to sustain life. [230]

Freebase nicotine reacts spontaneously with air and water, and as such it has to be produced and stored in an environment free of oxygen and water to prevent the spontaneous formation of niacin. The Britannica Encyclopaedia explains how to produce freebase nicotine:

> NICOTINE ($C_{10}H_{14}N_2$), an alkaloid, found with small quantities of nicotimine ($C_9H_{14}N_2$), nicoteine ($C_{10}H_{12}N_2$), and nicotelline, ($C_{10}H_8N_2$), in tobacco. The name is taken from Nicotiana, the tobacco plant, so called after Jean Nicot (1530-1600), French ambassador at Lisbon, who introduced tobacco into France in 1560. These four alkaloids exist in combination in tobacco chiefly as malates and citrates. The alkaloid is obtained from an aqueous extract of tobacco by distillation with slaked lime (calcium hydroxide), the distillate being acidified with oxalic acid, concentrated to a syrup and decomposed by potash (potassium hydroxide). The free base is extracted by ether and fractionated in a current of hydrogen. It is a colourless oil, which boils at 247°C. (745 mm.), and when pure is almost odourless. It has a sharp burning taste, and is very poisonous. It is very hygroscopic, dissolves readily in water, and rapidly undergoes oxidation on exposure to air. The free alkaloid is strongly laevo-rotatory. Its salts are dextro-rotatory. It behaves as a di-acid as well as a di-tertiary base.

Freebase nicotine does exist in tobacco leaves, in fact 'freebase nicotine' is simply the correct term for what we commonly just call 'nicotine'. Freebase nicotine is by no means an additive, rather it requires an alkaline environment to be released. As such, some tobacco companies add ammonia to the tobacco to ensure an alkaline environment is present which then allows the freebase nicotine to be released. This appears to negate Pankow's assertion that American Spirit has higher levels of nicotine than other brands like Marlboro. If certain brands did have higher yields of freebase nicotine and thus smokers became more addicted to them, then

---

[230] Cox, M; Lehninger, A.L; David, R; (2000) *Lehninger Principles of Biochemistry* Worth Publishers

those smokers would not feel satisfied by any other brands administering lower yields of nicotine. In fact, the entire freebase nicotine argument depends entirely upon the notion that smokers smoke solely, or at least primarily, for nicotine intake.

The majority of people nowadays, smokers and nonsmokers alike, have come to believe that smoking is an act of getting a nicotine hit into the body which then makes the smoker feel good, and believe that the primary reason that giving up smoking is so hard is because of nicotine withdrawal. This view of smoking and nicotine is not an old and accepted medical notion. It is a view that was officially rejected in the official Surgeon General Reports of 1964 and 1979, as shall be shown further into the chapter. Somehow, some people state that cigarettes are as addictive, or more addictive, than heroin and cocaine. This simply is not true. When a heroin or cocaine user gives up, they suffer severe physical withdrawal symptoms such as vomiting, nausea, diarrhoea, cramps, sweating and so forth. A smoker does not experience such symptoms. There is a difference between 'habit' and 'addiction': physical addiction is where a substance is needed for the body to function properly, hence a heroin user suffering horrible withdrawal symptoms – the drug has become needed for regular functioning. Smokers may be psychologically addicted, where they are duped into *believing* they need to smoke to function properly, but in reality abstaining from smoking will not result in the body breaking down. Furthermore, smokers tend to have a pattern to when they smoke e.g. first thing in the morning or after a meal etc, which is why it is hard to cease smoking – it is a daily habit with a particular routine; to break any habit is not easy.

The 1964 Surgeon General's Report validated the notion that smoking is habitual rather than an addiction:

> in medical and scientific terminology the practice should be labeled habituation to distinguish it clearly from addiction, since the biological effects of tobacco, like coffee and other caffeine-containing beverages, betel morsel chewing and the like, are not comparable to those produced by morphine, alcohol, barbiturates, and many other potent addicting drugs. (p 350)

Vincent-Riccardo Di Pierri PhD, author of *Rampant Antismoking Signifies Grave Danger*, notes that:

Cigarette smoking can also be understood as a habit if "habituation" is defined as the ease with which an activity becomes second-nature. Tobacco smoking is a simple action that becomes an extension of non-verbal activity. It can be practised in a multiplicity of circumstances for a multiplicity of reasons. As such, it can quickly become associated with strong cognitive, emotional and memory structures[231]

Page 351 of the 1964 Surgeon General's Report has definitions of a habit and an addiction, created by the World Health Organisation Committee on Drugs Liable to Produce Addiction. It defines addiction as:

a state of periodic or chronic intoxication produced by the repeated consumption of a drug (natural or synthetic). Its characteristics include:

1) An overpowering desire or need (compulsion) to continue taking the drug and to obtain it by any means;

2) A tendency to increase the dose;

3) A psychic (psychological) and generally a physical dependence on the effects of the drug;

4) Detrimental effect on the individual and on society

It then defines drug habituation as:

a condition resulting from the repeated consumption of a drug. Its characteristics include:

1) A desire (but not compulsion) to continue taking the drug for the sense of improved well-being which it engenders;

2) Little or no tendency to increase the dose;

3) Some degree of psychic dependence on the effect of the drug, but absence of the physical dependence and hence of an abstinence syndrome;

4) Detrimental effects, if any, primarily on the individual.

Don Oakley, in his book *Slow Burn: The Great American Antismoking Scam (And Why It Will Fail)*, provides a medical practitioners description of narcotic withdrawal. The symptoms he lists are

---

[231] Di-Pierri, V-R; (2003) *Rampant Antismoking Signifies Grave Danger: Materialism Out of Control* p171

"insomnia, marked anorexia, violent yawning, severe sneezing, weakness and depression, nausea and vomiting, intestinal spasm and diarrhea [sic]." He notes further symptoms of raised blood pressure and heart rate, along with the sufferer alternating between feeling very cold and sweating excessively. Oakley further describes the withdrawal process:

> The addict experiences waves of gooseflesh, his skin resembling that of a plucked turkey, which is the basis of the expression 'cold turkey'. Abdominal cramps and pains in the bones and muscles of the back and extremities are characteristic, as are muscle spasms and kicking movements that may be the basis for 'kicking the habit'... Occasionally, there is cardiovascular collapse.[232]

Such conditions never affect the abstaining smoker. As the 1964 Surgeon General's Report puts it "in contrast to drugs of addiction, withdrawal from tobacco never constitutes a threat to life." (p. 352)

So, what we realise now is that smoking is a habit, not an addiction, despite the 1988 Surgeon General's clearly redefining what it meant to be addicted to a substance – in a presumably deliberate and calculated manner to further the anti-smoking propaganda. It is no coincidence that the 1988 Surgeon General, C. Everett Koop, was a staunch anti-smoker (and one assumes he still is) and announced in 1984 the goal of making America "smoke-free" by the turn of the millennium. Evidently, such a goal was too ambitious and failed, but his successors are not letting a missed target dissuade them. Furthermore, Koop's reclassification of smoking as an addiction nicely coincided with the World Health Organisation's "5-year action plan: Smokefree Europe".[233] Thus, the seeds had been planted for a vision of a smoke(r)-free world, and those in authority would not let their unique positions miss the opportunity to put their stamp on the dream.

Besides the aforementioned explanation of nicotine, it is also important to remember that nicotine is largely burnt off when the tobacco is lit, so the average yield of a cigarette is 0.9 mg – less than a thousandth of a gram. Also, people pay a lot of money for

---

[232] Oakley, D; (1999) *Slow Burn, The Great American Antismoking Scam (And Why It Will Fail)* p.10

[233] Di-Pierri, V-R; (2003) *Rampant Antismoking Signifies Grave Danger: Materialism Out of Control* p.176

fine cigars, yet any cigar – and pipe – smoker will provide the same information: they smoke for the taste, aroma, and the general sensual pleasure of smoking. Cigar and pipe smokers seldom inhale, and Havana cigars contain only 2% nicotine – so if smoking tobacco was merely a way of getting nicotine into the blood stream, why would cigar smokers pay so much money for such little nicotine? The cigarette smokers who are not completely brainwashed into believing they are little more than nicotine addicts will also reveal that the pleasure they derive from smoking is multi-faceted – the taste and aroma, the feeling of the smoke in the mouth and throat, watching the smoke make patterns in the air, and the relaxing effect it has. It is a very ignorant opinion that smoking is just to fulfil a craving. As a matter of fact, in prisons where smoking is forbidden and access to tobacco is difficult, many inmates smoke corn silk and paper etc, which, of course, do not contain nicotine[234]. In *Smoke: A Global History of Smoking*, the author explains that "several letters, 'rolled like tobacco', were found on two Portuguese prisoners", highlighting that they smoked other materials when actual tobacco was unavailable. The truth of the matter is that smoking is a sensual pleasure that stimulates the taste buds, and allows the smoker to derive pleasure from the smell and hypnotic way the smoke seems to 'dance'.

Chris Holmes is a hypnotherapist who has aided thousands of smokers to give up, and he has recently authored a book entitled *Nicotine: The Drug That Never Was*.[235] In the book he explains why nicotine is not a drug at all, and is not the reason people smoke. Holmes is more than aware that smokers are not addicted to nicotine, but simply have a smoking habit. He says "nicotine does not qualify as a drug by any definition, and smokers' cravings (the urge to smoke) are completely unrelated to nicotine" and, in relation to the health industry claims that nicotine receptors go crazy when smokers go without a cigarette:

> In hypnotherapy we shut the cravings down,
> usually in a single session, proving all this bullshit about nicotine and 'nicotine receptors' WRONG. In the NRT ads, smokers are told that if they don't get nicotine, their nicotine receptors "go crazy" for nicotine... Oh, really?

---

[234] http://www.lcolby.com/b-chap11.htm

[235] http://www.truthwillout.co.uk/about/

Funny how that never happened to my smoking clients after hypnotherapy – they feel absolutely fine and normal, and I never mentioned 'nicotine receptors' once during the entire session.[236]

What Holmes is saying is what anyone who smokes or knows a smoker knows: that when a smoker does not smoke, their body does not give up on them, they do not break out in a cold sweat or start to vomit, they simply have cravings. We can have cravings for anything from sex to a hot dog, but we are not "addicted" to them, we merely know we enjoy them and wish to experience that pleasure again. As hedonistic creatures, it is our nature to seek pleasure and rewards. The fact that hypnotherapy works on smokers is proof alone that it is not a physical addiction, but a habit. After all, a heroin user may be hypnotised to no longer *want* heroin, but their body will still be letting them know it *needs* it.

Further proof of this is apparent when looking at nicotine patches and other such products. The small print of the products states that they only work with will power; it is an obvious point that smokers who give up without the products have will power anyway. If smoking was all about a nicotine hit then nicotine replacement in patches and gum would work well, yet the success rate has been shown to be just 1.6%.[237] These products work using a placebo effect: smokers believe they are addicted to nicotine, so believe nicotine replacement therapy will be effective. If nicotine was an addictive substance then putting them on a non-smoker when they slept would result in them becoming addicted to nicotine, yet this does not happen. Another overlooked point is that if nicotine were that addictive, all that would happen is people using nicotine patches and other products would simply become addicted to those instead, just as heroin users become addicted to morphine when they are given it on prescription to wean off the heroin. It must be stated here that there exist a small percentage of nicotine replacement therapy users who use it as though they are addicted. While people may claim this is indicative that nicotine is addictive, the truth is that it affects these people in the same way they believe smoking is addictive: a psychological addiction based in belief.

---

[236] From e-mail correspondence between Holmes and myself

[237] http://www.bmj.com/cgi/content/abstract/338/apr02_3/b1024

# Chapter 12: Government Health Warnings on Tobacco Products

> Many orthodox people speak as though it were the business of sceptics to disprove received dogmas rather than dogmatists to prove them. This is, of course, a mistake. If I were to suggest that between the Earth and Mars there is a china teapot revolving about the sun in an elliptical orbit, nobody would be able to disprove my assertion provided I were careful to add that the teapot is too small to be revealed even by our most powerful telescopes. But if I were to go on to say that, since my assertion cannot be disproved, it is intolerable presumption on the part of human reason to doubt it, I should rightly be thought to be talking nonsense.[238]

So spoke Bertrand Russell, a well respected philosopher. Whilst smoking has nothing to do with philosophy or flying teapots, the point he made most certainly does. What he is saying is that firstly, it is up to people with the claim to prove it, not those opposing the claim to disprove it, as a negative cannot be proved i.e. it cannot be proven smoking is *not* harmful, thus it is down to those who believe it *is* harmful to prove as much. Russell then makes an equally important point: just because something cannot be disproved does not instantly make the claim true. In other words, if someone like Stanton Glantz were to say "you cannot prove smoking or passive smoking is not harmful, therefore it is" then people would rightly tell him that is wrong. However, because the anti-smoking crusaders have built up an impressive catalogue to 'prove' smoking and passive smoking is harmful, everybody agrees that it is – despite the fact that hardly anyone of the public has actually read the studies, and despite the fact that they are entirely bogus.

More perplexing is that when scientists emerge and say they are bogus or smoking has not been solidly linked to disease, people get up in arms and protest about how ignorant that person is – but how would they know, without assessing the evidence for themselves? All they are doing is believing the side with the loudest voice.

---

[238] taken from Dawkins, R (2006) *The God Delusion* Black Swan Books

Many people believe that smoking is harmful otherwise there would not be warnings on the packets. Then again, there are plenty of other things without health warnings that perhaps should have them. For instance, cars do not come with a warning that a crash could paralyse or kill; junk food does not come with warnings of how it could damage health; alcohol, as of yet, does not have a warning stating the many problems abuse could lead to (though there are plans to get a government health warning on alcohol products).

What people are not so aware of is that the tobacco industry goes out of its way to encourage people to stop smoking, or state the risk involved. Philip Morris, the largest tobacco company in the USA, has its own Youth Smoking Prevention program, and on the website the company states how it tries to combat underage tobacco use.[239] The Philip Morris website also states they agree that smoking causes lung cancer, emphysema and heart disease, along with tobacco being highly addictive and that second-hand smoke poses a risk to people, despite these claims being highly questionable.[240] Furthermore, Philip Morris put warnings on their products in countries that do not require them to do so:

> We support a clear and consistent public health message about smoking, disease and addiction wherever we sell our products. We also support laws calling for cigarette manufacturers to place health warnings on cigarette packaging and advertisements. In countries where no such laws exist we voluntarily place warnings on our packs, cartons and adverts.[241]

The big question is 'why would a cigarette company want people to stop smoking?' Simple – the tobacco companies cannot prove smoking does *not* pose a threat to health, it is not possible to prove

---

[239]http://www.philipmorrisusa.com/en/cms/Responsibility/
Helping_Reduce_Underage_Tobacco_Use/Our_Approach/default.aspx?
src=top_nav

[240]http://www.philipmorrisusa.com/en/cms/Products/Cigarettes/Health_Issues/
default.aspx?src=top_nav

[241]http://www.philipmorrisinternational.com/PMINTL/pages/eng/smoking/
S_and_H.asp

a negative. For instance, if I post a letter and it does not arrive somewhere, the would-be recipient could not prove I did not send it. Even if I had not sent it they still could not prove it – I could have thrown it in the bin or never written it in the first place. However, a positive *can* be proven, so if the letter arrives, that is proof it was posted. In light of all the evidence smoking causes disease, whether or not that evidence can be disproved or not, it is not in the tobacco companies' interest to do so. In fact, they initially did deny the risk, but eventually realised that in doing so they had to work hard defending their products when they were sued. Nowadays, tobacco companies almost boast of the risk, they constantly state it and slap it on their products, and in countries where it is not required. Why? Because this way no one can turn around and say they did not know smoking was harmful for them. When a smoker gets lung cancer, they are likely to blame it on smoking, and thus blame the tobacco company. By putting a warning on, all the tobacco industry has to do is say 'you saw the warning and took the risk anyway, there is nothing we can do'.

The government health warnings did appear on tobacco products as government regulation, I am not for a moment suggesting that the tobacco companies one day decided to tell millions of people their products could kill them. The warnings surfaced as a result of the Surgeon General's Reports, and in America the warnings still state "Surgeon General's Warning". Despite court cases ruling that no animal study has succeeded in inducing lung cancer as a result of smoking, and Lord Nimmo stating that there is no evidence on an individual level that smoking causes lung cancer, the warnings still exist. These court cases highlight exactly why tobacco companies want warnings on their products: when the notion surfaced that smoking killed, a smoker who contracted disease could then sue the tobacco companies. However, with the warnings plastered all over tobacco products no smoker can say they did not know of the risks of smoking, they knew the risks, saw the warnings and the responsibility of their actions lie squarely on themselves.

# Chapter 13: Health Benefits of Smoking

Perhaps one of the best ways we can see the evidence of how there is a political agenda against smoking is by realising that we are to believe it is the only natural substance to have no medicinal properties. Despite the ongoing battle to combat underage and binge drinking, there is still a lot of publicity about the health benefits of one or two drinks per day. Yet, we are never told of any beneficial properties of tobacco despite the fact that it was used for medicinal purposes by American Indians for millennia to treat wounds and swellings and other ailments such as coughs and colds.

There is a large body of evidence detailing the health benefits of smoking. A 1990 book by M. Castro states that a homeopathic remedy can be cultivated from the dry leaves which is used in the treatment of nausea and travel sickness.[242] Another book [243] speaks of how tobacco leaves can be applied to the skin to treat rheumatic swelling, skin diseases and scorpion stings. Yet another publication[244] mentions tobacco has a long history of being used by medical herbalists as a relaxant, as well as the leaves being antispasmodic, discutient, diuretic, emetic, expectorant, sedative and sialagogue.

Edgar Cayce, a famous psychic healer, recommended smoking four to six all-tobacco cigarettes each day for people who suffer from asthma. A member of the alt.smokers discussion group, whose name will be withheld for confidentiality, is an asthma sufferer and she finds that smoking cigarettes soothes her lungs and relieves the attacks. It has been known for centuries that smoking is a remedy for a cough or bad throat, and whilst many smokers abstain from smoking while they have an illness, those who do smoke with a sore throat often notice it feels better.

As mentioned in chapter eleven, it has been known for quite some time that smokers have far lower rates of Parkinson's disease

---

[242] Castro. M. (1990) *The Complete Homeopathy Handbook.* Macmillan. London.

[243] Chopra. R. N., Nayar. S. L. and Chopra. I. C; *(*1986) *Glossary of Indian Medicinal Plants (Including the Supplement).* Council of Scientific and Industrial Research, New Delhi.

[244] Grieve; (1984) *A Modern Herbal.* Penguin

212

and Alzheimer's disease, and studies show that smoke contains monoamine oxidase inhibitors (MAOIs) which are used in treatment of Parkinson's. In the March 20th 2007 edition of *Science News*, Megan Rauscher wrote of a study showing that there is a temporal relationship between smoking and reduced risk of Parkinson's disease – the study found the protective effect wanes after smokers give up.[245] The study was published in the March 6th 2007 edition of *Neurology*, and researcher Evan Thacker, from Harvard School of Public Health, stated:

> It is not our intent to promote smoking as a protective measure against Parkinson's disease. Obviously smoking has a multitude of negative consequences. Rather, we did this study to try to encourage other scientists…to consider the possibility that neuroprotective chemicals may be present in tobacco leaves.

As has been stated previously, it adds more validity to a study when the researchers seem surprised by their findings. In this case, whilst the researchers do not necessarily seem perplexed, they make it apparent that they believe smoking is harmful, so they are in no way trying to conduct a pro-smoking study.

The study consisted of Thacker and colleagues analysing data, including detailed lifetime smoking histories from 79,977 women and 63,348 men participating in the Cancer Prevention Study II Nutrition Cohort. Of the nine years of follow-up, 413 subjects developed definite or probable Parkinson's disease.

It was found that people who had never smoked had a 'normal' risk of Parkinson's disease, compared with ex-smokers having a 22% lower risk and current smokers having a 73% lower risk. In ex-smokers, it was found that the longer they had smoked, and the longer the duration they had smoked (i.e. the more cigarettes per day coupled with a longer overall duration) related to a decreased risk of Parkinson's disease. The researchers stated:

> A 30% to 60% decreased risk of Parkinson's disease was apparent for smoking as early as 15 to 24 years before symptom onset, but not for smoking 25 or more years before onset.

They also noted that they were not alone in this finding:

---

[245] http://www.data-yard.net/10v2/parkinson.htm

The results were similar for men and women, and were also similar to the results of studies by many other researchers looking at the same topic.

FORCES have compiled a list of studies which have linked Parkinson's disease with non-smokers, which is available on their website.[246]

Smoking also seems to protect against Alzheimer's disease and, as with Parkinson's, FORCES have compiled an extensive list of independent studies examining the link between smoking and Alzheimer's. They have largely concluded that smoking is beneficial in protecting oneself from the onset of the disease, and that list is viewable online also.[247] It is well known that smoking helps to improve concentration and mental ability, so it is perhaps this effect on the brain that permits smoking to protect from Alzheimer's. Appel put forth the idea after noting that of thirty patients, twenty-four of them had never smoked in their lives. Subsequently, there have been nineteen case control studies published, and they are the ones on the aforementioned FORCES list. There was a clear negative association from the studies, with fifteen of the nineteen studies reporting a lower risk of Alzheimer's disease in men and women who smoked or had previously smoked. Of the remaining four, none found an increased risk of Alzheimer's in smokers.

A reanalysis by a researcher called Graves found that:

> A statistically significant inverse relation between smoking and Alzheimer's disease was observed at all levels of analysis, with a trend towards decreasing risk with increasing consumption ($p=0.0003$). A propensity towards a stronger inverse relation was observed among patients with a positive family history of dementia.

A very interesting Dutch study, entitled "Apolipoprotein E Genotype and Association Between Smoking and Early Onset Alzheimer's Disease"[248] found that smoking can reduce the risk of

---

[246] http://www.forces.org/evidence/carol/carol36.htm

[247] http://www.forces.org/evidence/carol/carol16.htm

[248] http://www.ncbi.nlm.nih.gov/pubmed/7703749?dopt=AbstractPlus

Alzheimer's tenfold – more than any other drug or other treatment. The results found:

> The inverse association between smoking history and early onset Alzheimer's disease could not be explained by a decrease in the frequency of the apolipoprotein e4 allele. Among carriers of this allele with a family history of dementia subjects with a history of smoking had a strongly reduced risk of early onset Alzheimer's disease (odds ratio 0.10 (95% confidence interval 0.01 to 0.87)).

The researchers concluded:

> The results suggest that the inverse relation between smoking history and early onset Alzheimer's disease cannot be explained by an increased mortality in carriers of the apolipoprotein e4 allele who smoke. The association is strongly modified by the presence of the apolipoprotein e4 allele as well as by a family history of dementia.

Mentioned in chapter five was how Doll found smokers who inhale suffer less lung cancer than non-inhalers, hinting to a protective effect. Also shown was how various animal studies, as well as the WHO's passive smoking study, confirm this. Surprisingly, there are more studies validating this. The Multiple Risk Factor Intervention Trial (MRFIT), with over 12,000 participating males including over 8,000 smokers, put the participants into two groups: special intervention (SI) and usual care (UC), with the SI group being encouraged to stop smoking and take up 'healthier' lifestyle habits, and the UC group doing what they would normally do. The conclusion reads:

> None of the hypotheses proposed to explain the unexpected higher rates of lung cancer mortality among SI as compared with UC subjects were sustained by the data.[249]

In other words, the SI group, who were told to stop smoking, had more lung cancer sufferers than the UC group who continued to smoke. Actually, the SI group had 22% more lung cancer.

There are plenty of scientists who have reported on the apparent paradox of smokers suffering less lung cancer, including: Axelson & Associates (Scandinavian Journal of Environmental Health 41:46 1978), Dahlgren (Lakartidingen 76:4811 1979), Weiss

---

[249] http://works.bepress.com/ockenej/157/

(Journal of Occupational Medicine 18:194 1976 and 22,527 1980), Pinto and Associates (Archives of Environmental Health 33:325 1978). The general consensus on these findings is that tobacco smoking promotes mucous formation, which acts as a protective coating in the lungs which can, in turn, prevent carcinogenic particles penetrating the lung tissue – as shown in the study with mice and radiation. It is also this mucous production that encourages smokers to cough; so, then, smokers cough is not, as perceived, harmful and the sign of ill health but rather a beneficial act which helps rid the body of toxins and protects smokers from respiratory illness (a German study also confirms this, which we will see further into this chapter).

One very interesting study, published in *Circulation,* noted that, concerning restenosis (the occlusion of coronary arteries), smokers are more likely to survive, heal and do well. The study was relatively large, with 8,671 participants. The researchers concluded:

> In patients undergoing contemporary PCI, cigarette smoking is associated with a lower rate of subsequent TLR without affecting angiographic restenosis. These findings have important implications for the follow-up of smokers after PCI and suggest that cross-study comparisons of rates of clinical restenosis must account for the potential confounding effect of smoking.[250]

Another study, conducted by Dr. Christopher Heeschen of Stanford University, found that:

> simple plant protein, nicotine, applied in small harmless doses, produced new blood vessel growth around blocked arteries to oxygen-starved tissue. The research, involving animal studies, showed that the nicotine agent created more new blood vessels in blocked arteries than any other known growth factor. The new agent could be used to treat failing hearts and limbs with poor circulation. It holds the potential for non-surgical heart by-pass procedures.[251]

Whilst it is stated that the medicinal application does not come from smoking, this is not the same as saying it *cannot* come from smoking. In other words, they are not advocating smoking but it

---

[250] http://www.data-yard.net/34/circulation_2001_104_773.htm

[251] http://www.data-yard.net/10/toben.htm

will have the same benefits. As shown in chapter five, numerous studies have shown that nicotine stimulates vascular growth, which is in keeping with the results of this study. [252] [253] [254]

A small study that is worth mentioning found that, despite conventional wisdom, smokers are at lower risk for gum recession. Researchers in Germany said that the present data does not support the hypothesis that smokers are at greater risk for gum recession – which is interesting as numerous warnings on tobacco products state smoking can cause gum disease and recession. The study, entitled "Gingival Recession in Smokers and Non-Smokers with Minimal Periodontal Disease" was published in the 2002 *Journal of Clinic Periodontology.* Sixty-one systematically healthy volunteers aged nineteen to thrty took part. Of the participants, thirty smoked twenty or more cigarettes a day, and the remaining thirty-one were non-smokers. At the start of the study, about half of both groups had receding gums at one or more sites. The research showed that non-smokers had three times more severe gum recession of over two millimetres than in smokers (23% non-smokers compared to 7% smokers). It was found that smoking status did not influence the risk of recession after statistical adjustments for various factors were made. The factors included periodontal probing depth, recession at baseline, how often the volunteers brushed their teeth, gender, tooth type and the site of disease. Naturally, with such an incredibly small sample size the results must be taken with caution, but it is an interesting finding that merits a follow-up.

Whilst it is true to say this is a very small study, and it only used people already suffering from periodontal disease, it is still worth mentioning. The reason for this is if smoking really did increase the risk, then we could expect to see at least a slight increase of risk, or, given the sample size, an equal risk to non-

---

[252] http://ajp.amjpathol.org/cgi/content/abstract/160/2/413

[253] http://www3.interscience.wiley.com/journal/104541376/abstract

[254] http://jap.physiology.org/cgi/content/abstract/84/6/2089

http://www.docguide.com/news/content.nsf/PaperFrameSet?
OpenForm&id=48dde4a73e09a969852568880078c249&newsid=8525697700
573E1885256B89005D6A9E&u=http://www.blackwell-synergy.com/servlet/
useragent?func=synergy&synergyAction=showAbstract&doi=10.1034/j.
1600-051x.2002.290207.x&ref=/news/content.nsf/news/
8525697700573E1885256B89005D6A9E

smokers, but the findings showed a three-time risk increase in non-smokers, which suggests that smoking is not a risk factor. Furthermore, what is even more noteworthy is that the researchers stated at the outset that current information – what the warnings on packets are based on – does not support the hypothesis that smoking is a risk factor, in other words such warnings on tobacco products should not be there as it remains unproven.

Interestingly, there are at least some studies showing smoking may be beneficial during pregnancy – and certainly is not a risky activity. One such study shows that smoking is associated with a *reduced* risk of hypertension during pregnancy[255] with the researchers stating:

> Smoking is associated with a reduced risk of hypertension during pregnancy. The protective effect appears to continue even after cessation of smoking.

Another study on smoking and pregnancy, conducted by Lain et al in 1998, found that smokers had a reduced risk of developing preeclampsia. This is not a new discovery, a family friend of mine is a nurse and the hospital she worked in ran a study on smoking and pregnancy many years ago. They found the same results: women who smoked were at less risk of preeclampsia. Of course, the information was not divulged because it is politically correct to only release information of the negative effects of tobacco, not the objective view. It is quite worrying that an agenda and the corruptness of organisations come before the wellbeing of many millions of people.

There is also evidence that smokers are less likely to develop endometrial cancer. One study, by William T. Creasman MD et al, found that:

- Smoking apparently decreases the risk of developing endometrial cancer.
- The effects of smoking are related to body weight. Heavier women who smoke have the greatest reduction in risk.
- Women who smoke are known to undergo menopause 1-2 years earlier than women who do not smoke.[256]

---

[255] http://www.data-yard.net/2/14/ajog2.htm

[256] http://emedicine.medscape.com/article/254083-overview

Another study on the subject, published at National Center for Biotechnology Information, found that:

> both current and past smoking are associated with a lower risk of endometrial cancer. The findings provide insight into disease etiology and suggest that the influence of smoking on endometrial cancer risk occurs even in early adulthood, is long-lasting, and may not be attributed solely to short-term hormonal modulation[257]

A third study, from China, found the same thing. The results were featured in an article on Reuters,[258] and the principal investigator Dr. Bin Wang of Nanjing Medical University said that "The benefit of smoking was observed almost exclusively in postmenopausal women and not in premenopausal women"

Wang and his colleagues investigated their research by collecting data from thirty-four previous studies published through June 2007, and their findings, which appear in the *American Journal of Medicine*, show that current and former smokers were at a decreased risk of between 18-29%. Further to this, Wang and his colleagues found that women on hormone replacement therapy (HRT) who smoked were around 50% less likely to contract endometrial cancer than their non-smoking counterparts.

Another interesting benefit of smoking appears to be that osteoarthritis is reduced threefold in smokers. A study conducted by A. Samanta et al, published in the *Oxford Journals*,[259] looked at whether osteoarthritis in women is affected by hormone levels or smoking and concluded that the "study demonstrates no association between oestrogen-related hormonal events and OA, but a negative association between smoking and LJOA" (LJOA being large joint osteoarthritis).

Yet another apparent benefit is the internal antioxidant SOD (superoxide dismutase) is doubled in smokers, and a recent article labels the higher SOD "the elixir of eternal life" based on

---

[257] http://www.ncbi.nlm.nih.gov/pubmed/15645490

[258] http://uk.reuters.com/article/healthNews/idUKCOL56218920080715

[259] http://rheumatology.oxfordjournals.org/cgi/content/abstract/32/5/366

animal experiments.[260] Apparently SODs mop up free radicals which are linked with ageing.

There is a theoretical physicist who regularly posts on forums such as speakeasy.com under the name 'Nightlight', and who has conducted huge amounts of research looking at the hard science of smoking. (S)he comments on smokers having a reduced MAOI B enzyme – with smokers in their sixties having MAOI B enzyme levels of people in their twenties. Most interestingly, this is not the result of nicotine but another, as yet unknown, compound within tobacco.[261] A pharmaceutical drug named Deprenyl became very popular in life-expansion circles and it mimics the MAOI B inhibition of tobacco smoke, as well as being used in treatment of Parkinson's and Alzheimer's. The theoretical physicist goes on to say how long term tobacco smoking also blocks the peripheral MAOI B also by almost halving its levels, thus keeping organs decades younger from middle age; and then shows photos of a 122 year old smoker Jeanne Louise Calment and ninety year old chain-smoker Deng Xiaoping. Also posted on the forum link are photo scans of a smoker and non-smokers body, comparing the MAOI B levels. I strongly suggest to all readers to have a look at the forum and read the wealth of information for themselves.[262]

The same theoretical physicist also speaks of how glutathione, the body's chief antioxidant and metal detoxifier, as well as many other antioxidants and detoxifiers, are strengthened with smoking and provides a link to a study which I have also referenced.[263] The study found that:

> Compared with nonsmokers, cigarette smokers had 80% higher levels of ELF total glutathione, 98% of which was in the reduced form

---

[260] http://www.telegraph.co.uk/news/uknews/1550409/Scientists-find-elixir-of-eternal-life---in-a-worm.html

[261] http://www.nida.nih.gov/NIDA_Notes/NNVol13N3/tobacco.html

[262] http://speakeasyforum.com/eve/forums/a/tpc/f/173601742/m/2391082291?r=3071036391#3071036391

[263] http://jap.physiology.org/cgi/content/abstract/63/1/152?ijkey=3ea8cff64c6d72a42e1d4ef7cf9f6fd2485e5921&keytype2=tf_ipsecsha

The study showed that smoking twenty to thirty cigarettes on a daily basis affects the immune system in a way that twenty to thirty exercise breaks throughout a day would affect the muscles. After just a few weeks of such exercise, gains in muscle size and strength would be noticeable.

Many people reject any notion that smoking can have positive effects because they experience a decrease in lung function – or, at least, *believe* they are experiencing such a decrease. In reality, this 'breathlessness' is caused by excess mucous production, stimulated by smoking, hence 'smoker's cough'. This is not a bad thing, in fact it is quite the opposite – by increasing mucous production, the body is then excreting various toxins from the lungs, and the mucous layer adds protection against harmful, penetrating toxins or carcinogens. In very recent history, the Royal College of Physicians of London promoted smoking for its health benefits and smoking was actually compulsory in elite schools with one Eton student recollecting that he "was never whipped so much in his life as he was one morning for not smoking."[264] The Semai people of Malaysia are actually encouraged to start smoking at age two, before they can even talk. All personal ethics aside, this does serve irreplaceable as a case study, for if smoking lowered lung capacity and so forth, the Semai people would be all but useless by about age twenty. However, Dr. C. Y. Caldwell examined 12,000 people, including chest X-rays, to determine what effects this habit of lifelong smoking was doing to them. Their paper, printed on February 26th 1977 in the BMJ, stated that of the 12,000 Semai examined, there was not a single case of lung cancer.[265]

It is also known that smoking doubles the levels of the vital detox enzyme catalyse which neutralises alcohol, cyanide, formaldehyde and toxic metals.[266] The study examined the activities of superoxide dismutase (SOD), catalyse (CAT), and glutathione peroxidase (GSHPx), in alveolar macrophages (AM) from cigarette smokers and from smoke-exposed hamsters. They found that "the activities of SOD and CAT from AM of smokers and smoke-

---

[264] http://members.iinet.com.au/~ray/TSSOASb.html

[265] http://tobaccodocuments.org/landman/507927406-7466.html?zoom=750&ocr_position=above_foramatted&start_page=51

[266] http://www.ncbi.nlm.nih.gov/pubmed/2310098?dopt=Citation

exposed hamsters were twice that found in control subjects (p less than 0.01)."

The benefits of smoking are not unknown – in fact, the pharmaceutical industry is quietly trying to develop drugs to mimic the positive actions of tobacco smoke. A pharmaceutical industry funded group Society for Research on Nicotine and Tobacco (SRNT) has released a brief review of the neuroprotective aspects of smoking. It is very telling that SRNT are trying to mimic tobacco whilst admitting on their home page that they are striving "for the prevention and treatment of tobacco use."[267] There are no prizes for working out that "treatment" is just a way of saying 'stop smoking, use our wonder drugs instead'.

The review itself says:

there is evidence to suggest that these agents may be useful in preventing or treating a wide variety of central nervous system (CNS) disorders, including:
* Parkinson's disease
* Alzheimer's disease
* attention deficit/hyperactivity disorder, and possibly Tourette's syndrome;

other conditions for which nicotinic agents could theoretically be helpful include:
* obesity
* depression and
* anxiety.

In addition to its effects on CNS disorders and functioning, cigarette smoke seems to exert a protective or beneficial influence on some

* immunological and
* inflammatory disorders and on certain
* hormone-related and
* reproductive problems.

---

[267] http://www.srnt.org/

as well as admitting there is an "inverse association between cigarette smoking and a variety of disorders". On Attention Deficit Hyperactivity Disorder the review says

> Nicotine administration has been shown to improve attentiveness, and nicotine also promotes the release of dopamine as does current pharmacologic treatments of ADHD. A study by Levin and colleagues showed significant reduction in reaction time, reaction time variability, and increased accuracy on several cognitive tasks with nicotine administration in 11 adults diagnosed with ADHD. Additionally, these subjects rated themselves as having significantly more vigor than when they were administered placebo. Further studies are continuing with chronic administration. Currently used treatments, methylphenidate, amphetamine and pemoline have this mechanism of action.

On schizophrenia:

> Nearly 90% of schizophrenics smoke. One possible explanation for this phenomenon is that schizophrenics may smoke in part because nicotine may improve their ability to filter out and ignore irrelevant sensory information, which may be related to an impairment of inhibitory mechanisms which act to decrease attention to repeated stimuli (sensory gating).

It is a very interesting point that of the 90% of smoking schizophrenics, most are chain smokers and they suffer 30-50% less cancer, both lung and other sites, than non-smokers of the same age. [268]

On immunological and inflammatory disorders:

> Cigarette smoking seems to impair several aspects of immune functioning, including T-cell functioning and antibody response;40 consequently, a benefit for immunologically-mediated disorders is conceivable.

---

[268] http://www.schres-journal.com/article/PIIS0920996404002130/abstract

Inflammatory bowel disease:

> Illustrative of the diversity of sites of nicotine's action in the body is preliminary evidence of a potential role in inflammatory bowel disease. Silverstein reported several cases which linked cessation of cigarette smoking to the onset of inflammatory bowel disease, and/or symptom improvement with nicotine administration via nicotine gum. These studies show that current smokers have a reduced risk and former smokers had a slightly increased risk of being diagnosed with ulcerative colitis (UC) and that the risk of onset of UC appears to be substantially increased shortly after quitting smoking. Initial clinical trials of the addition of nicotine gum to standard treatment in UC have shown improvement in about 50% of patients. A study of 6-week treatment with nicotine patches has also shown significant improvements in global clinical and histological appearance, severity of symptoms, and remissions.

Aphthous ulcers:

> A protective effect of cigarette smoking or smokeless tobacco use and the risk of recurrent aphthous ulceration of the mouth has emerged in several studies, though not in all. Some investigators have published case reports noting a worsening of the ulcers after smoking cessation, with relief after resumption. These effects may be due to the increased oral keratinization associated with tobacco use; the possible efficacy of nicotine chewing gum suggests that nicotine is an active moiety.

Extrinsic allergic alveolitis:

> Smoking is clearly inversely related to extrinsic allergic alveolitis (farmers' lung, pigeon breeders' lung), a chronic immunologically-mediated lung disorder. In addition to a lower risk of the clinical syndrome itself, smokers have lower levels of the serum antibodies associated with the disorder.

So there we have it, the pharmaceutical industry is well aware of the benefits of tobacco smoking and is now dedicating time and money to trying to mimic the properties so they can generate large income for themselves. They are telling people not to smoke as it is so harmful, whilst simultaneously singing of what amazing benefits it actually has.

A 1999 study found that smokers suffer less respiratory illnesses than their non-smoking counterparts.[269] The study compared seventy-five workers in an aluminium pot room, with twenty-three never smokers, thirty-eight current smokers and fourteen former smokers, with fifty-six controls in the same plant. The controls were watchmen, craftsmen, office workers, laboratory employees, with eighteen non-smokers, twenty-one current smokers and seventeen ex-smokers. The results showed that

> Smokers in the potroom group had a lower prevalence of respiratory symptoms than never smokers or ex-smokers, which was significant for wheezing (2.6% v 17.4% and 28.6% respectively, both p <0.01)

and "in potroom workers, impairment of lung function due to occupational exposure was found only in non-smokers."

William Whitby, author of the *Smoking Scare De-Bunked*, wrote in 1986:

> In my medical practice patients frequently told me that smoking relieved their coughs. Because this was contrary to what the text books and the lecturers said, I at first thought they just imagined it. But as it continued over the years I began to wonder if there was something in it. My own experience with smoking showed me just how right they were. From childhood I had a history of bronchitis accompanied by marked wheezing. I was warned by doctors not to smoke. In my late thirties I got such frequent disabling attacks, sometimes with pneumonia, that they seriously interfered with my work and made life rather distressing. An old country doctor said to me one day, "I used to be like you. Then someone put me on to the secret – take up the pipe. I did and I've never been better." I had

---

[269] http://oem.bmj.com/cgi/content/abstract/56/7/468

never smoked because of warnings from chest 'experts' but remembering my patients' claims, I took the old doctor's advice. The change in my health was miraculous. In the years since I took up smoking, my chest troubles have been few. It is many years since I have had an attack of bronchitis. I am sure I would have been dead long ago if I hadn't smoked. When I hear 'experts' talking or I read books decrying smoking in chest conditions I just smile and think how little they know.

A short but very interesting little point is that coenzyme Q10 – the supplement raved about in new beauty products – is extracted from the tobacco leaf. Coenzyme Q10 is ubiquitous, in that it is present in each and every one of the cells in our bodies. However, the source which has it in most abundance is the tobacco leaf. Perhaps it can be shown that smokers who have a healthy lifestyle have younger looking skin than healthy-living non-smokers.

A final point to consider is that in seventeenth century England schoolteachers encouraged children to take their pipes and tobacco to school, presumably as it helped with concentration of the students. In many far eastern countries women smoke cigars, even the children smoke and everybody thinks it is a good thing. The aforementioned Semai people are prime examples of tobacco being a cultural staple.

It is evident, as this chapter has shown, that there is plenty of evidence that tobacco as a product and being smoked has numerous benefits and health-promoting qualities. Moreover, the evidence gathered is not from the tobacco industry or from groups with vested interests in tobacco consumption, but independent studies that were published in respected journals. Such results highlight the bias within the smoking politics; if objectivity were the order of the day then the health organisations, along with the government, would provide all the available information. It is apparent, however, that they cherry pick data to present to the public.

This chapter will conclude with quotes and conclusions of various studies on various benefits of smoking and nicotine.

In human studies, reported performance improvements with post-trial administration of nicotine have all involved associated learning (Mangan and Golding 1883; Colrain et all 1992; Warburton et al 1992)…Nicotine improves

226

performance by increasing the attentional resources available for such strategic processing[270]

1. Nicotine improves attention in a wide variety of tasks in healthy volunteers. 2. Nicotine improves immediate and longer-term memory in healthy volunteers. 3. Nicotine improves attention in patients with probable Alzheimer's Disease[271]

Researchers observed lessening of tic frequency and severity 3 minutes after subjects chewed [nicotine] gum, even more so at 10 minutes[272]

In humans, nicotine-induced improvement of rapid information processing is particularly well documented... Preliminary studies have found that some aspects of the cognitive deficit in Alzheimer's disease can be attenuated by nicotine[273]

Improvement in attention, learning, reaction time, and problem solving have been reported...Different processes, including attention, stimulus evaluation, and response selection, appear to be involved in the effect of nicotine on human information processing[274]

Despite the absence of change in memory functioning, these results demonstrate that DAT [Alzheimer's disease]

---

[270] Rusted JM et al; (1992) *Facilitation of Memory by Post-Trial Administration of Nicotine: Evidence for Attentional Explanation* Psychopharmacology

[271] Warburton D.M. (1992) *Nicotine as a Cognitive Enhancer* Progress in Neuro-Psychopharmacology and Biological Psychiatry

[272] Rickards E. H; (1992) *Nicotine gum in Tourette's disorder* American Journal of Psychiatry. Note: the subjects were all children suffering from Tourette's.

[273] Levin E.D. (1992) *Nicotinic Systems and Cognitive Function* Psychopharmacology

[274] Le Houzec J; Benowitz N.L. (1991) *Basic and Clinical Psychopharmacology of Nicotine* Clinics in Chest Medicine

patients have significant perceptual and visual attentional deficits which are improved by nicotine administration[275]

"When you look at people who smoke, and people who don't smoke...you find those who smoke cigarettes are about half as likely to get Parkinson's disease."[276] (Quote by Dr David Morens of the University of Hawaii School of Public Health. Dr Morens and colleagues examined 34 studies on smoking and Parkinson's, the study was published in the June '95 issue of *Neurology*.)

> The influence of smoking on the risk of developing ulcerative colitis is well documented. Compared with lifetime nonsmokers, the risk is reduced in smokers...[277]

> When association between cigarette smoking and UC [ulcerative colitis] are examined, never-smokers are approximately three times more likely to develop UC than smokers. A consistent finding from study to study is that quitters have a mildly increased risk of UC which suggests that cigarette smoking may have a protective effect [278]

> It is beyond doubt that smokers are protected against ulcerative colitis, and the more that is smoked the greater the protection – so those on 25 cigarettes a day or more have a risk as little as one-tenth that of non-smokers[279]

## The World's Oldest People

In society today, we are constantly told – and never allowed to forget – that smokers are statistically more likely to get a variety of

---

[275] Jones, G.M.; Shakian, B.J. et al; (1992) *Effects of Acute Subcutaneous Nicotine on Attention, Information Processing and Short-Term Memory in Alzheimer's disease* Psychopharmacology

[276] Field, R *Stunned docs discover cigarettes stop Parkinson's* 15/06/1995 issue of New York Post

[277] Tysk, C; Jarnerot, G. (1992) *Has smoking changed the epidemiology of ulcerative colitis* Scandinavian Journal of Gastroenterology, June issue

[278] Lashner, B.A.; (1992) *Inflammatory bowel disease: family patterns and risk factors"* Comprehensive Therapy

[279] Dr Martin Osbourne, surgeon at the Royal Free Hospital in London, quoted in the 7/9/1993 issue of the *Daily Telegraph*

diseases than non-smokers, and accordingly have a lower life expectancy than non-smokers. This book has shown that the link between smoking and disease is unproven and a weak argument. The figures are grossly adjusted or exaggerated at best, and completely fabricated at worst. Studies are paid for by anti-smoking organisations who profit or otherwise benefit from smoking being blamed for cancer and other diseases, such as funding from nicotine replacement therapy manufacturers. True science uses animal studies as a basis for health effects on humans, and the sweetener aspartame was used as a prime example in chapter two. Tobacco has never once caused lung cancer in *any* animal, meaning that we are supposed to believe only humans are negatively affected by smoking. Furthermore, the anti-smoking movement would have us believe that tobacco is the only natural product that has no benefit whatsoever – it is a product which only brings harm. This is simply not true, and many studies and quotes from physicians and doctors show this. What becomes apparent is that the notion that smoking causes illness and premature death is one of the biggest lies ever told; whether its origins were more genuine, albeit misguided, is irrespective, as the anti-smoking movement has long since left science behind, and intentionally so.

Given this, it is no surprise that the "other" statistics i.e. the ones that contradict the ones made up to show smoking is harmful, are not released. After all, it is one thing saying that smokers die younger, but where are the facts? Who is raising the point that, actually, a very large percentage of the elderly population smoke, and smoke heavily? Who is raising the point that the life expectancy has been increasing steadily for a very long time, despite, at one point, the majority of the adult population being smokers? And the fact that cigar and pipe smokers tend to be elderly, and tend to outlive non-smokers? Apparently, not many people make these points. The ones who do are ignored, or shouted down. Any sensible and half-intelligent person would question this – after all, if the anti-smoking crusaders are so convinced they are right, and have so much evidence to back up their claims, they would not need to shout loudly or adjust figures or hide other figures as the truth would speak for itself.

The truth does speak for itself. The truth just does not get heard enough, because the truth states that smoking does not cause illnesses or premature death. Most of the people who lived to be the oldest people on record happened to be smokers.

The first person is Zhang Shuqing. On May 7th 2007, Zhang turned 100, as reported in *China Daily*[280] and he began smoking and drinking strong liquor in his early twenties. Since he started, Zhang has smoked every day and had a drink with every meal, and his grandson claims that Zhang has smoked over a ton of tobacco in his lifetime. Not only did Zhang live to be over 100 years old, he was also in good health for his birthday – not only was he living, but he was not fighting against lung cancer or struggling to breathe as a result of emphysema.

On August 28th 2006, ABC News reported on the world's oldest man: a 115 year old Puerto Rican named Emiliano Mercado del Toro.[281] When the United States seized Puerto Rico from Spain in 1898, Emiliano was six years old. We are also told that he smoked for seventy-six years, quitting at the age of ninety. It is interesting to note that here is a man who started at fourteen and smoked for seventy-six years. Furthermore, when Emiliano started smoking, there were no filters. If he started smoking in 1916, aged fourteen, he would not have smoked a filtered cigarette until the 1950s or 1960s, meaning he smoked for forty or fifty years without a filter – something we are told helped lower the rates of smoke-induced lung cancer.

On Monday 24th February 2003, FOX News ran an article on the longest living American: John McMorran of Lakeland, who lived to be 113.[282] He smoked cigars, drank beer and ate greasy food, eventually giving up smoking at ninety-seven years of age. As with Emiliano, McMorran was in good health until he died of heart problems related to pneumonia. His great-granddaughter Lisa Saxton told FOX that "he was never sick". Apparently, John McMorran smoked until he was ninety-seven, lived until he was 113, and did not have any problems from his smoking habits.

In early 2003, the Italian newspaper *Libero* reported updates on the Tobacco Massacre of Milan (it is unclear whether the reporter was being sarcastic with the title, or if s/he was just ignorant to what the facts mean). The city has a population of 2.2 million, with two being over 110, five being 109 and twelve being

---

[280] http://www.data-yard.net/10b3/100_smoker.pdf

[281] http://www.data-yard.net/10m2/oldest.htm

[282] http://www.data-yard.net/10a1/oldest.htm

106. 217 of them are just 100 years old, 167 are 101, and 115 are 102 years old. Further to this, 35,000 Milanese are aged between eighty-five and ninety-four, with a further 92,000 being between seventy-five and eighty-four. The paper also reports that the overwhelming majority smoke, drink, or eat fatty foods, and most do all three. Some of the Milanese have even smoked for over ninety-four years. What is particularly interesting about this article is that it is not about just one or two individuals, but thousands of people who lived to old age and smoked. Not something that can be passed off as luck or good fortune.

One of the most famous elderly smokers was the Queen Mother, who liked to smoke cigarettes and drink gin cocktails. She died peacefully in her sleep aged 101 and, aside from suffering from a cold, was in good health.

Keeping in line with the famous elderly smokers, Billy Wilder, director of *Some Like it Hot* amongst other classics, died aged ninety-five of pneumonia and was a lifelong smoker.

Milton Berle died aged ninety-three from colon cancer. The *San Francisco Chronicle* featured an article on March 28th 2002 on his death,[283] and one paragraph stated

> His trademark cigar rarely left his hand. In an interview two years ago, Berle said he'd smoked cigars since he was 12. "I figure if George Burns can smoke 20 cigars a day his whole life and live to be 100, why should I worry if they're bad for me?"

The *New York Times*, 1st December 1999, ran an article on John Berry, a stage and movie director. Berry smoked a pipe and died aged eighty-two. Whilst this is not seen as incredibly old by today's standards, it is above the life expectancy and older than many would expect a smoker to live to.

On September 9 1999, the *Montreal Gazette* featured the 100th birthday of Isabella Gibson, who smoked for most of her life. Whilst she gave up, she also said that on the day of her 100th birthday "I smoke when my son gives me one, it feels good."

Wenceslao Moreno, better known as Senor Wences, appeared as a ventriloquist numerous times on the *Ed Sullivan Show*. The April 20th 1999 issue of *The Washington Post* had an article on

---

[283] http://www.data-yard.net/10n/berle.htm

Wences,[284] where we are told he died aged 103 and smoked for most of his life, even on television with his puppets.

The world's oldest woman, Jeanne Calment, died aged 122. She began smoking as a young woman but gave up at the age of 117 because she had gone blind and was too proud to ask someone to light her cigarette often. She started smoking again when she was 118 because not smoking made her miserable.[285]

Marie-Louise Meilleur of Canada died aged 116. She chain-smoked all her adult life, with her grandson saying "she always had a cigarette dangling from her lips as she worked", as reported in the *Miami Herald*, 15th August 1997. She stopped smoking when she was almost 100, although we would be told that she was lucky to smoke and live that long.

One of the world's oldest men was Christian Mortensen, who was featured in the *San Francisco Chronicle* on 5th August 1997, in an article entitled "114 and Still Smoking". Mortensen had smoked cigars for most of his life, and at the age of 114 was still smoking. I am not sure if he ever stopped, or what age he died, but 114 is an incredibly long time to live – in fact, at the time of the article, he was said to be the longest living man in the world.

George Cook was Britain's oldest man and he died in his sleep aged 108. *Houston Chronicle*, 29th September 1997, stated that he "smoked heavily for 85 years before giving up tobacco at the age of 97"

*The Scottish Daily Record*, 15th December 1997 issue, ran an article on Ivy Leighton who was aged 100 at the time. She smoked a pack a day for eighty-five years, cutting down after she reached a century.

Finally, there are two men who claimed to be the world's oldest living humans, but their dates of birth cannot be certified. The first is Ali Mohammed Hussein of Lebanon, who featured on CNN on 13th May 1997. Hussein claimed to be 135 and he "smokes like a chimney." The second is Narayan Chaudhari, a Nepalese who claims to be 141. He says the secret of him living such a long life is "raw tobacco and no alcohol". His story was featured in *Nando net, Agence France-Press*, under the heading "Nepalese man claims to be 141, which would make him world's oldest" on 12th February 1998.

---

[284] http://www.forces.org/articles/files/ventriloq.htm

[285] *USA Today* 18th October 1995

Despite these people all living to ages that most people think unfathomable, most will be categorised as a smoking-related death. Any person who smokes, regardless of their age or cause of death, goes down as another statistic of death by smoking. In this way, the crusaders can produce extremely large numbers to show how fatal smoking is – even if non-smokers die of the same cause (and not forgetting these figures are lumped in with the estimated smoking-related deaths explained in chapter six). Apparently anti-smokers forget that despite there being fewer smokers now than there used to be, the longest life expectancy in the world is only around eighty years old, so the previous examples show that smokers are perfectly capable of reaching a ripe old age – and, indeed, outlive non-smokers in far higher numbers than can be attributed to luck.

Many anti-smokers will put these people down to being lucky, but there is safety in numbers and the city of Milan alone should repel this notion, and smokers holding the longevity records should be the final nail in the coffin.

# Chapter 14: Past Attacks on Smoking

A common misconception is that the war on smoking we are currently experiencing is a result of the scientific discovery that smoking is harmful, and that it is to protect the health of the public. What people are not aware of, though, is that this is not the first time in history smoking has been targeted. Chapter five mentioned how the Nazis banned smoking and tried linking it to cancer, but this was not the first attack either.

Ever since smoking was introduced there have been people who despise it. There have been those who dislike the smell, or find second-hand smoke irritating. There are those who believe that inhaling smoke *must* be harmful and thus hate it, and there are those who simply hate it for no real reason. Truth be told, there have been people who hated smoking from day one. Christopher Columbus himself was one such person. When he and his crew, Rodrigo de Jerez and Luis de Torres, reached Cuba in 1492 his crew tried smoking the pipe whilst Columbus spoke against it, even referring to his crew as descending to the level of "savages" and wrote that "it was not within their power to refrain from indulging in the habit". It was his crew, de Jerez and de Torres, who put tobacco on their boat to take to Europe, thus introducing it to the Europeans for the first time. Instantly, people hated it just as much as others loved it, and the Catholic Church considered it ungodly and heretical as it was a plant of the godless 'Red Indians'.

The 1600s were a time of smoking regulation: in Russia first-time offenders were whipped, had their noses slit, and were sent to Siberia; second-time offenders were executed. In Turkey, under the rule of Sultan Murad IV, smokers were castrated for their habit and up to eighteen smokers a day were being executed, whilst Chinese smokers were killed by decapitation. In 1900 Washington, Iowa, Tennessee and North Dakota outlawed the sale of cigarettes, and in 1901 there was strong anti-tobacco activity in forty-three of forty-five American states:

> only Wyoming and Louisiana had paid no attentionn to the cigarette controversy, while the other forty-three states either already had anti-cigarette laws on the books, were considering new or tougher anti-cigarette laws, or were the scenes of heavy anti-cigarette activity. (Dillow, 1981:10).

In 1904 in New York City, a woman was sent to prison for smoking in front of her children; and in the same city in the same year another woman was arrested for smoking in her car with the arresting officer stating "you can't do that on Fifth Avenue". In 1905 in Indiana a legislative bribery attempt was exposed, leading to a passage of a total cigarette ban. In 1907 business owners refused to hire cigarette smokers, with the August 8th *New York Times* stating "business…is doing what all the anti-cigarette specialists can't do". The list goes on, but the point has been made that the attacks on smoking now are nothing new.

In 1917 there was a similar attack against smoking as there is now. I am not sure if it is surprising or not that the tactics are the same – on the one hand it is surprising because the methods were used and eventually failed, but on the other hand when there is no supporting evidence to the theory there is only so much that can be said. In the 1917 attack, the focus was on children, much the same as it is today. Another similarity is that doctors were 'informing' people that smokers were likely to get, or certainly going to get, tuberculosis, "tobacco heart", and blindness. During this time, surgeons asked patients whether or not they smoked as part of the preparation of surgery, just like they do now (dentists even ask now, because supposedly smokers need a different anaesthetic to non-smokers), and insurance companies asked prospective clients whether they smoked. By 1927, the attack had passed and people were smoking again without any worries or fear.

A magazine entitled *The Instructor*, August 28th 1917 issue, was billed as "the annual anti-tobacco issue". The cover featured a picture of President Woodrow Wilson, with the caption "Woodrow Wilson – a National Example – the President Does Not Smoke" (a very eerie precursor to that of the Nazis proclaiming that the Fuhrer Hitler does not smoke). It is with no doubt that if the authors of the magazine knew that Wilson were to suffer a stroke that left him debilitated less than a year after the magazine was published they would not have chosen to have him on the front. The magazine featured articles and cartoons with the intention of demonising tobacco and smoking, which are included in the appendices of this book.

The first excerpt in the appendices is an article that is clearly nothing but sheer propaganda. It starts by attempting to show smoking as harmful with nothing but weak logic:

> If the use of tobacco is not injurious, WHY does the life insurance company wish to know whether the applicant smokes? WHY does the surgeon, contemplating a serious

operation, ask whether the patient smokes? WHY are athletes, in training, forbidden to smoke?

Then it becomes even more ridiculous:

> WHY do cigarette smokers make the vast majority of mistakes in bookkeeping? WHY do none of the books which deal with the principles of success in life, and give advice to young men of ambition, advice the use of the cigarette? WHY is it that youthful criminals are almost invariably smokers?

The article attempts to show smoking is harmful because statistically smokers supposedly make mistakes in bookkeeping, and books giving advice on lifestyle do not offer smoking as a recommendation. This is dubious to say the least; there is nothing of any scientific note to be found anywhere. The article then goes on to imply that smoking rots the brain:

> One puff does not destroy the brain or heart; but it leaves a stain, and every other puff deepens that stain, until finally the brain loses its normality, and the victim is taken to the hospital for the insane or laid in a grave. One puff did not paralyse the young man in the wheel chair; but the many puffs that came as a result of the first puff, did. The telltale stains on the fingers were indicative of the deep stains made upon the nerve cells…One puff did not destroy his obedient, helpful spirit; but many puffs made him a disobedient, dishonest boy

Excerpt two in the appendices is just as ridiculous. "It has been scientifically proved that smoking produces grave effects on mind, body and soul". Actually, the soul itself has not been proven to exist, and we certainly have no information to know what benefits and harms it. This tactic of persuasive language ("proven") is one still used by the anti-smoking movement to entice people to believe they are correct in their statements. This excerpt then goes on to quote a doctor, who rambles on about how smoking causes vertigo, indigestion, and hand tremors. If this was all really proven almost a hundred years ago, then it is with no doubt that Stanton Glantz and co. would have no trouble in reminding us of this, and there would be piles of studies to back it up. In actuality, these so-called facts are nothing more than mindless drivel and propaganda intended to convince people smoking is wrong. The article has a huge picture in the middle of it, with one road called 'success' and another called 'failure', on the road to success is one non-smoking male, and the failure road has three smokers, all looking very miserable indeed (p282 of this book). It is things like this that really point out the agenda going on – that drawings and false claims are needed to put people off highlights that no scientific data exists.

The other excerpts are much the same so I will not go over all of them; they are included at the end of the book. This magazine tells us a lot, and whilst it is sad that we are suffering the same bogus attack now as we were in 1917, with the same tactics and lies, it is uplifting to note that the original attack failed and this one is doomed to do just the same.

Perhaps the only difference between past attacks and the current attack is that this one has a seemingly limitless supply of money, allowing the claims and 'research' to continue growing. When the public are told that something other people do affects them personally, they go up in arms and this has furthered the anti-smoking movement by giving success to the claims of second-hand smoke being harmful. This would be more tolerable if smoking was on an equal playing field, and cars were fitted with a top speed of much lower than what they have in an attempt to prevent speeding and the resultant deaths, or a ban on alcohol in public places to prevent drunken attacks, but this is not the case. To clarify this point, the above examples are not being advocated by myself, but are rather pointing out the hypocrisy of targeting only one substance or product. If others were included, the draconian rules would at least be universal.

The war on smoking has reached heights never seen before, to the point where in summer 2007 the leaders of the Californian town Belmont were debating a bill which proposed to ban smoking on every street, park and pavement, as well as all homes except detached houses. As if this were not enough, any person witnessing a smoker breaking this rule and not reporting it to the police would be punishable as it would be illegal to not report it. The most baffling part of this bill is that outside air has all the fumes from vehicles to worry about, so the premise appears to be that cigarette smoke is more hazardous to health than constant exposure to petrol and diesel fumes. Thankfully, it did not pass, although there are now places in North America where smoking outdoors is prohibited. With regards to the ban in houses, as if the second-hand smoke myth was not ridiculous enough, are we now to believe that tobacco smoke permeates its way through walls and ceilings to kill our neighbours too? The very idea of this is nothing short of crazy, and ridiculously portrays tobacco smoke to be on par with a deranged serial killer who hunts out his victims.

Anti-smokers are nothing new. In fact, they have not even thought of a new mantra to the ones from the times of tobacco being first introduced, as King James I wrote in his book *A Counter Blaste To Tobacco*, "loathsome to the eye, hateful to the nose, harmful to the brain, dangerous to the lungs." There was, like today, no such scientific basis for any claims, and we now know that cancer and pollution turn organs black, not smoking. In the same time period, anti-smokers claimed that smokers' brains were 'sooty', as smokers were reminiscent of chimney sweeps. Of course, not even anti-smoking extremist Stanton Glantz would claim that smokers have soot on their brains. Quite simply, there have always been, and will always be, people who loath smoking. The main reason for this is simply intolerance and the tired excuse of 'not wanting to be subjected to your smoke' failing to remember, of course, that each and every day we are subjected to things we dislike or have no choice over, such as car fumes, polluted food and water, pesticides on food, loud music, and so on. We have no choice if we drive perfectly sensibly yet someone crashes into the back of our car. Conversely, in today's society everyone has the choice to avoid tobacco smoke. Aside from the blanket ban, smoking has been banned on all forms of public transport for many years, in addition to shops, offices, cinemas and so forth. There were also non-smoking pubs for those who preferred to frequent them. Moreover, modern technology makes it possible to have clean air in an enclosed area that permits smoking. Apparently, though, this is not good enough and *all* buildings need to be smoke free so that non-smokers can go wherever they please without any discomfort. To top it off, and in keeping with the ostracisation of smokers, anti-smokers say it is *smokers* who are selfish and uncaring towards the needs of others.

# Chapter 15: The Pharmaceutical Connection

As said in the opening of the previous chapter, most people believe that this war on smoking is for the health of the public and the result of scientific evidence. What is becoming more and more well known, however, is that the pharmaceutical companies are very much pulling the strings on the matter for their own personal gain, and are no strangers to using trickery to sell their products.

Every pharmacy, and indeed many shops, has a huge display of smoking-cessation products such as gum, patches or the inhaler. Who makes these products? The pharmaceutical industry. Who buys them? Smokers trying to give up or smokers unable to smoke at work or in a travel situation like an aeroplane. Put two and two together and we get this result: the pharmaceutical industry has direct interests in people trying to stop smoking as a large percentage of those people will go and buy smoking cessation products. Each time there is a no-smoking day compliant smokers will turn to nicotine products as they have been told an addiction is the reason why they smoke, and this turns a profit for Big Pharma.

The anti-smoking mantra is preached everywhere, even in schools to young children who will then go home and nag their parents to stop smoking. Everywhere we turn there is something negative said about smoking, smokers are now forced to huddle outside buildings to smoke, it is not politically incorrect to shout abuse at smokers yet it is forbidden to shout abuse at virtually any other well defined group such as obese people or gay people. More and more, smokers are becoming the outcasts of society, becoming little more than men in the stocks for the almighty public to walk by and spit on for their crimes. All this prompts smokers to give up their habit, but the campaigns have been so successful that smokers no longer believe they have a habit, but rather an addiction which requires the help of a doctor. Compliantly the smoker wanders down to his doctor to get prescribed a nicotine replacement, or he goes to his pharmacy for the same product, but either way he is putting money in the pocket of Big Pharma.

There are very tell-tale quotes from the annual reports of pharmaceutical companies, and the following is from the 2001 report of Pharmacia Corporation, the company who make Nicorette:

> Driving the growth of Consumer Healthcare is one of the world's top 10 otc [over the counter] brands: the Nicorette

family of smoking cessation products. Nicorette showed renewed vitality last year with sales of **$299 million, up 37 percent** over the prior year. Among the highlights of 2001 were the highly successful September otc launch of Nicorette in Japan (the first otc smoking cessation product to be approved in that country); the reacquisition of sales and marketing rights to Nicorette gum in Canada; and the launch of a new **global marketing campaign**. Nicorette currently **controls about half of the worldwide smoking cessation market**.[286] [Emphasis mine]

The emphasis in the above quote is mine to show the driving force of the stop-smoking campaign. One product alone in 2000 generated revenue of $299 million, which was over a third more than the preceding year. Since 2001 the anti-smoking war has increased, and no doubt the revenue for Pharmacia Corporation has too. The quote mentions Japan, Canada, and the global marketing campaign, so we will look at those three in more detail.

In the same time period as the report there have been stringent anti-smoking laws applied in Japan, despite the fact it is a country that is usually very tolerant of smoking. It is now forbidden to smoke in the streets and there are very severe crackdowns. It is no coincidence that this happened right at the same time Nicorette began to be pushed in Japan.

Canada now has very harsh anti-smoking laws and outlooks, and in one year there was $480 million public Canadian dollars spent by the ministry of health for a "total war" against smokers, including the removal of parental authority of smokers who refuse to stop (the removal of parental authority has been evidenced in courts for many years in child custody battles with a smoking parent). In 2003 there was a hearing which would have lead to the criminalisation of tobacco, resulting in the pharmaceutical industry having total control over nicotine. Whilst on the issue of Canada and the pharmaceutical industry, in 2008 the Canadian health minister proposed proposition C51, which would make all natural supplements and herbs illegal and only obtainable with a prescription. A similar bill failed in Australia a few years ago, and whether the bill will pass or not has yet to be seen but it certainly

---

[286] http://media.corporate-ir.net/media_files/NYS/PHA/reports/ar2001.pdf

serves as a great example of the power and corruption of Big Pharma.

Finally, the global marketing campaign. In 2002 the World Health Organisation tried to get an international treaty to beat tobacco globally.[287] According to the WHO website, 'the fifth session of the Inter-governmental Negotiating Body (INB, October 14-25) will examine a new text of the Framework Convention on Tobacco Control (FCTC) that proposes options culled out of four years of negotiations. WHO Director-General, Dr. Gro Harlem Brundtland, said:

> this is a critical moment for the negotiations. The technical work is complete and I believe the time has come for countries to show their determination about curbing the tobacco epidemic.

Whilst people rarely think of the world scene and instead believe their country happens to be working at the same time as other countries in banning tobacco because it is so harmful, the truth is the countries are all doing it at the same time for political reasons – and at the same time as Big Pharma marketing its relevant products.

Page ten of the 2001 annual report of Glaxo Smith Kline,[288] the manufacturers of smoking-cessation pill Zyban, tells us about the competition that they face:

> In the USA, the major competitor products in over-the-counter (OTC) medicines are: … private label smoking cessation products. In the UK the major competitor products are … Nicotinell (smoking cessation remedy).

This point is continued on page sixty-one:

> Smoking control sales declined eight per cent, reflecting competition in the US market following the introduction of private label Nicotine Replacement Therapy (NRT) gum and patch. The introduction of two new GlaxoSmithKline smoking control products in the US market, Clear NicoDerm Patch and Nicorette Orange Gum, prevented

---

[287] http://www.who.int/mediacentre/news/releases/pr78/en/index.html

[288] http://www.gsk.com/financial/reports/ar2001/annual-report-01/ GSK_Report.pdf

further inroads from private label brands. Excluding the USA, smoking control sales grew by 58 per cent.

What this quote tells us is that due to competition in America leading to a loss of 8%, Glaxo Smith Kline released a further two products which then allowed their sales to grow by 58%.

On page forty-six the report says that Zyban was released in France. Only a year later, in 2002, the National Anti-Smoking Committee in France produced a film which showed an emaciated forty-nine year old male lung cancer victim dying, filmed five days before his death. The film was used in a television campaign to prompt people to stop smoking – which would, in turn, drive up the sales of the newly released Zyban.

On page forty-nine the report gives us the sales of Zyban for 2001: £337 million, or $440 U.S. dollars. This is a staggering number yet it is a decrease from the £375 million of 2000. Whilst they do not say why the decrease is there, it is undoubtedly due to two things: 1) the competition of other brands, and, most importantly, 2) the product received negative publicity for it being linked to causing heart attacks in smokers using the product. There is also the fact that it simply does not work – nicotine replacement therapy (NRT) has a failure rate of over 98%. However, many smokers try to give up smoking using a nicotine replacement product, fail, and try again at another time. This may be a deliberate act on the pharmaceutical industry's behalf; after all, they know as well as anyone that nicotine is not the reason people choose to smoke and so they know that the smoker will keep buying the products for many years each time they try to give up.

Page fifty-eight tells us that:

> In the smoking cessation market, Zyban's growth of **54 per cent** reflected its rollout into European markets following European Union approval in April 2000. Initial sales were particularly strong in the UK and Germany [emphasis mine]

It is apparent that banning smoking in public places is completely imperative to entice people to stop smoking and start using these products instead. These reports tell us that just two smoking cessation products have grossed about $670 million in just one single year, and this is without being the largest of all pharmaceutical companies – that accolade goes to Johnson & Johnson.

Johnson & Johnson uses its philanthropic arm, the Robert Wood Johnson Foundation, to be a very generous financer of anti-smoking studies and activists, and in the USA in the past ten years has financed roughly half a billion dollars to the cause, including to Karen Lewis of the World Health Organisation's Tobacco Free Initiative, almost $100 million to the Smokeless States initiative, and $84 million to the Centre for Tobacco-Free Kids. Wanda Hamilton has compiled a list of all the organisations funded by RWJF, which is available online,[289] as well as a very extensive list of anti-tobacco researchers and activists who are funded by RWJF.[290]

Indeed, the monetary donations are not merely acts of generosity, but are more along the lines of investments: donate money to an anti-smoking organisation, and drive up sales of smoking-cessation products. And while RWJF focuses mainly on the USA, Glaxo Smith Kline and Pfizer are working the global scene, with both companies being paid-up members of the aforementioned Tobacco Free Initiative. Not ones to leave all their eggs in one basket though, they also partly funded the Institute for Global Tobacco Control and fund the UK's Roy Castle Foundation. Pfizer also gave $33 million to ASH International, a newly formed group.

If this is not convincing enough, the Tobacco Control journal published an article in 2005 entitled "Toward a comprehensive long term nicotine policy" in which the authors stated that "The immediate need is to capture all nicotine into a regulatory system." That regulatory system is nicotine manufactured and dispensed solely by the pharmaceutical industry. Still unconvinced? The Centre for Tobacco-Free Kids are currently demanding the American government to reduce the nicotine levels within cigarettes to zero, and the authors of the above article also state that nicotine in the regulatory system should be in "more outlets, including vending machines" and at "reduced prices". They continue further, saying "tobacco availability should become progressively less easy" until the time comes when, instead of cigarettes, nicotine replacement from the pharmaceutical industry becomes "the dominant source of the drug".

---

[289] http://www.forces.org/evidence/money/listorg.htm

[290] http://www.forces.org/evidence/money/antipro.htm

The clear vision then is the ultimate goal of the pharmaceutical industry as the sole creators and distributors of nicotine, and one can just imagine what the profits would be if they are already so huge when people can still obtain it in tobacco products.

What is most unsettling is that this current anti-smoking movement has the money and power to see their aims through. Limitless funds and people in high places will always be helpful to the group(s) lucky enough to have them, and the following quotes serve to highlight how powerful the pharmaceutical industry is:

The top 10 drug companies are reported to have profits averaging about 30 percent of revenues-a stunning margin. Over the past few years, the pharmaceutical industry as a whole has been by far the most profitable industry in the United States.[291]

In every year since 1982, the drug industry has been the most profitable in the United States, according to Fortune magazine's rankings. During this time, the drug industry's returns on revenue (profit as a percent of sales) have averaged about three times the average for all other industries represented in the Fortune 500.[292]

Put together, the market capitalization of the four largest [pharmaceutical] companies is more than the economy of India.[293]

The truth becomes very apparent that the health establishment has become very close to Big Pharma, an industry which now puts huge amounts of money into anti-smoking studies and activists in return for the health minister of each country banning smoking in public

---

[291] Angell, M. June 22nd 2000 *The Pharmaceutical Industry – To Whom Is It Accountable?* New England Journal of Medicine

[292] Public Citizen Report July 23rd 2001 *Rx R&D Myths: The Case Against the Drug Industry's R&D 'Scare Card'*

[293] David Earnshaw, formerly director of European government affairs for SmithKline Beecham, now leader of Oxfam's campaign on access to medicines. Quoted in Roger Dobson. April 28, 200"*Drug Company Lobbyist Joins Oxfam's Cheap Drugs Campaign,*" BMJ, 322, 1, p. 1011.

which then drives up the sales of products to aid smoking cessation. We now live in an era where medicines and pharmaceutical drugs are the norm, and we feel we cannot live without them – to take them away will force us back to a time when people were riddled with infections and disease and died far too young.

However, pharmaceutical companies lie to us on a daily basis. They create new illnesses or exaggerate existing ones in an attempt to sell more drugs.[294] According to one study,[295] pharmaceutical companies have spent more money lobbying Congress in America than any health care organisation. Actually, Big Pharma spends almost twice as much money on marketing as on research,[296] and two thirds of drugs claimed to be new are either identical or slightly modified versions of existing drugs.[297]

This would be more acceptable if the drugs worked, but they are often unnecessary and can be extremely dangerous. Indeed, an article in *Discover* in September 2006 explains that vultures in India are dying due to residues of the anti-inflammatory drug Voltaren that they ingest when they eat dead cattle carcasses. In fact, western medicine is between the first and third leading cause of death in the United States; some sources say heart disease and cancer are the top two, and others say smoking is number one. Barbara Starfield M.D., in the *Journal of the American Medical Association* July 26th 2000, cites 12,000 deaths per year to unnecessary surgery, 7,000 deaths annually to medication errors in hospital, 20,000 annual deaths in hospitals to other errors, and 80,000 deaths per year to infections contracted in hospitals. Finally, she says there are 106,000 deaths per year due to the negative effects of drugs, totalling 225,000 deaths per year – putting it in third place.

---

[294] *Washington Post* May 30 2006 The article focuses on "disease mongering" where a symptom that would normally be considered a normal part of life is labelled as a disease that requires a drug to treat it. Examples include: shy people who think they have "social phobia"; high strung boys who are diagnosed with attention deficit disorder; people with slightly elevated blood pressure who have "pre-hypertension"

[295] http://www.eurekalert.org/pub_releases/2004-03/cwru-dca032304.php

[296] *Nursing Online Education Database* March 27 2008

[297] Ibid

A point made in Dr Mercola's[298] September 14th 2006 newsletter is that the death rate actually decreases when doctors go on strike.

Gary Null PhD et al released a paper in October 2003 entitled "Death by Medicine", part of which is included below:

> A definitive review and close reading of medical peer-review journals, and government health statistics shows that American medicine frequently causes more harm than good. The number of people having in-hospital, adverse drug reactions (ADR) to prescribed medicine is 2.2 million. Dr. Richard Besser, of the CDC, in 1995, said the number of unnecessary antibiotics prescribed annually for viral infections was 20 million. Dr. Besser, in 2003, now refers to tens of millions of unnecessary antibiotics. The number of unnecessary medical and surgical procedures performed annually is 7.5 million. The number of people exposed to unnecessary hospitalization annually is 8.9 million. *The total number of iatrogenic deaths shown in the following table is 783,936.* **It is evident that the American medical system is the leading cause of death and injury in the United States.** The 2001 heart disease annual death rate is 699,697; the annual cancer death rate, 553,251.*[299]* [Emphasis mine]

It is disturbing to think that the industry to which we literally entrust with our lives is responsible for killing so many people, and are at best the third leading cause of death in America, or at worst the number one leading cause of death. This same industry is trying very hard to demonise smokers in an attempt to sell its own products, and people believe it is an honest move from scientific evidence that smoking is harmful.

---

[298] www.mercola.com

[299] Null, G et al; (2003) *Death By Medicine* Nutrition Institute of America

# Chapter 16: The Cancer Research Institutes

It has been noted numerous times in this book that various cancer charities, such as the American Cancer Society, fund anti-smoking studies, as do heart charities like the British Heart Foundation. To many, this would appear to be inconsequential. It is likely that the majority of the population believe the cancer charities are simply wonderful organisations providing a great service to people. However, the reality is that these organisations are as involved as the pharmaceutical companies.

A little known fact is that over the years there have been many scientists who have developed methods of curing cancer, many of them having degrees of success. Perhaps the two most notable doctors in the cancer field are Otto Warburg and Johanna Budwig.

The former was the son of physicist Emil Warburg and one of the twentieth century's leading cell biologists.[300] He gained degrees in Chemistry and Medicine in 1906 and 1911 respectively. His special interest lay in investigating vital processes by physical and chemical methods, which led to him attempting to relate such processes to phenomena of the inorganic world. He conducted detailed studies on the assimilation of carbon dioxide in plants, the metabolism of tumours and the chemical constituent of the oxygen transferring respiratory ferment. Later in his career he discovered that the flavins and nicotinamide were the active groups of the hydrogen-transferring enzymes which, coupled with the iron-oxygenase discovered previously, gave a complete account for the oxidations and reductions in the living world. For this, he was awarded a Nobel Prize in 1931. The discovery also opened up the fields of study into cellular metabolism and cellular respiration, allowing him to show that cancerous cells can live and develop in the absence of oxygen.[301]

In 1924, Warburg hypothesised that cancer is caused by the fact that tumour cells mainly generate energy by non-oxidative

---

[300] Krebs, H.A; (Nov., 1972). "Otto Heinrich Warburg. 1883-1970". *Biographical Memoirs of Fellows of the Royal Society* (The Royal Society) **18**: 628–699.

[301] http://nobelprize.org/nobel_prizes/medicine/laureates/1931/warburg-bio.html

breakdown of glucose, as opposed to healthy cells generating energy from oxidative breakdown of pyruyate. Pyruyate is an end-product of glycolysis and is oxidised with mitochondria. This led Warburg to state that cancer should be seen as a mitochondrial dysfunction:

> Cancer, above all other diseases, has countless secondary causes. But, even for cancer, there is only one prime cause. Summarized in a few words, the prime cause of cancer is the replacement of the respiration of oxygen in normal body cells by a fermentation of sugar[302]

Warburg carried on developing the hypothesis and held prominent lectures to outline both the theory and the data.[303] Furthermore, although not being considered the cause of cancer, the notion that cancer cells change to glycolysis is now widely accepted. According to J Kim, some people have suggested that this discovery could be used to develop anticancer drugs.[304] In addition, cancer cell glycolysis has been used as the foundation of positron emission tomography, which is a medical imaging technology that relies solely on this phenomenon.[305] It is interesting to note that his findings were not applied in any natural sense, but instead were considered for drugs i.e. making profit.

The importance of Otto Warburg's discoveries cannot be overstated or emphasised enough. So amazing were they, in fact, that an Otto Warburg Medal has been in existence since 1963. Awarded by the German Society for Biochemistry and Molecular Biology, it honours and encourages pioneering achievements in biochemical and molecular biological research. So prestigious is the

---

[302] Warburg, O.H. *The Prime Cause and Prevention of Cancer* accessed October 30, 2007

[303] Warburg O. H. (1956) *On the origin of cancer cells* Science 123 (3191): 309–14

[304] Kim JW, Dang CV (2006). *Cancer's molecular sweet tooth and the Warburg effect.* Cancer Res. 66 (18): 8927–30

[305] Som P, Atkins HL, Bandoypadhyay D, *et al.* 1980. *A fluorinated glucose analog, 2-fluoro-2-deoxy-D-glucose (F-18): nontoxic tracer for rapid tumor detection.* J. Nucl. Med. 21 (7): 670–5

medal that it is the highest award for biochemists and molecular biologists in Germany.

The latter researcher, Dr Johanna Budwig, was also a biochemist. She was an expert on fats and nutrition and essentially followed on where Warburg left off. As a precursor to the following description, Budwig was nominated seven times for the Nobel Prize.

During her extensive research, Dr Budwig made a number of remarkable discoveries. Firstly, people seriously ill with cancer always had low levels of phosphatides and lipoproteins in their blood, whilst healthy people had both compounds in normal amounts. Secondly, most cancer patients' blood contained a green-yellow substance, indicating lower levels of haemoglobin than normal. This prompted her to theorise this is why cancer patients are often anaemic and weak. Finally, she discovered that the blood of a healthy person contains much higher levels of Omega-3 essential fatty acids (EFAs) than that of cancer patients. She said in a speech in Zurich, 1959:

> Without these fatty acids, the respiratory enzymes cannot function and the person suffocates, even when he is given oxygen-rich air. A deficiency in these highly unsaturated fatty-acids impairs many vital functions. First of all, it decreases the person's supply of available oxygen. We cannot survive without air and food; nor can we survive without these fatty acids. That has been proven long ago.[306]

And in one her 1994 book on the medicinal qualities of flax oil she said:

> I often take very sick cancer patients away from hospital where they are said to have only a few days left to live, or perhaps only a few hours. This is mostly accompanied by very good results. The very first thing which these patients and their families tell me is that, in the hospital, it was said that they could no longer urinate or produce bowel movements. They suffered from dry coughing without being able to bring up any mucous. Everything was blocked.

---

[306] November 2, 1959 in Zurich, Switzerland

It greatly encourages them when suddenly, in all these symptoms, the surface-active fats, with their wealth of electrons, start reactivating the vital functions and the patient immediately begins to feel better.

She also later came to the conclusion that much of the disease and chronic illness facing the western world today is caused by poor nutrition and processed foods and oils. Perhaps we can see the evidence of this around us, with almost every item in a shop containing processed vegetable oil and the majority of those in the western world having an excess of Omega-6 and deficiency of Omega-3 fatty acids. This may explain why Ernst Wynder's research showed that the lighter smoking American's suffered higher rates of lung cancer than the heavier smoking, healthier-eating Japanese. There is a wealth of testimony supporting the effectiveness of Budwig's diet,[307] with the notable one being from Dr Dan C. Roehm M.D. FACP, an oncologist and former cardiologist, who said "This diet is far and away the most successful anti-cancer diet in the world"

There is a family-run website that has a lot of information on the effectiveness of Budwig's diet.[308] The family had first-hand experience with it after one member was diagnosed with cancer and saw remarkable recovery following Budwig's plan. Budwig herself had over 1,000 documented successes (and perhaps many more undocumented ones) but her research was suppressed. In 1991 Budwig was on the cover of *Alive* magazine, which was reporting on her death. The article within explained that at the hands of the cancer research institutes she lost her job, her laboratory, and her privilege to publish academically. She did, however, triumph in over thirty court cases.[309] She recounted that:

> the *Zentralausschuss für Krebsforschung* [Central Committee for Cancer Research] in Germany, represented by three professors, tried to take legal action against me, for just this statement I have made before you, the presiding judge said:

---

[307] http://www.healingcancernaturally.com/budwig_protocol.html#Quotes

[308] www.beckwithfamily.com

[309] http://www.encognitive.com/files/Dr.%20Johanna%20Budwig, %20a%20remarkable%20scientist.pdf

"Doctor Budwig's documents and papers are conclusive. There would be a scandal in the scientific world, because the public would certainly support Doctor Budwig." He advised the professors to withdraw their accusations but they were obstinate and did not comply. Then even the University's Chancellor, himself a jurist, became involved. The entire case was declared null and void in order to avoid a public outcry.[310]

Thus, we are left with a degree of evidence of causes and treatments of cancer. Yet these findings and treatments are never mentioned by our doctors or the media. Apparently the reason for this lies in the fact that money cannot be made off the back of them, because the necessary products can be purchased cheaply at various stores. In other words, no expensive prescriptions or radiotherapy and no large pay cheque for any cancer institute or pharmaceutical company.

This can be validated by the fact that the Kanzius machine has been hailed as the future of cancer treatment. On July 20th 2008, CBS News reported the story of John Kanzius, a man with no medical background whatsoever who developed a possible cure for cancer – in his kitchen, with his wife's cooking pans.[311] Kanzius was a retired businessman and radio technician, and used that experience to develop a radio-wave emitting machine to target and destroy cancer cells. CBS stated in the report that if clinical trials go well then:

> the Kanzius machine will zap cancer cells all through your body without the need for drugs or surgery and without side effects. None at all. At least that's the idea.

Idea, indeed. The claim that the machine will have no side effects comes from Kanzius himself, whose only actual testing comes from putting his hand into the radio signal field – akin to someone having a line of cocaine and then saying it is harmless because no

---

[310] http://www.healingcancernaturally.com/guidesandbooks2.html

[311] http://www.cbsnews.com/stories/2008/04/10/60minutes/main4006951.shtml

immediate harm is apparent. The side-effects may only occur after exposure to high levels of the radio-waves.

The treatment is much more than mere radio-waves, though. Kanzius knew that high-powered radio waves cause metal to heat up, leading him to wonder what would happen if a tumour was injected with metal and then hit with radio-waves.

The machine has been picked-up by two major research centres: the University of Pittsburgh and M.D. Anderson. A liver cancer surgeon, Dr Steven Curley, is testing it at the latter centre and believes it is the "most exciting thing that I've encountered" in twenty years of research. The most probable reason for this excitement is the fact that Kanzius' idea permits, perhaps even *requires*, the use of nanoparticles. Nanoparticles are a modern invention of science; miniscule carbon or metal particles, so small that thousands can fit into a single cancer cell. Being metallic, they can be injected into a cancer cell and zapped with Kanzius' machine.

As wonderful as this all sounds, some perspective is needed. Dr Mercola stated in a May 10th 2008 article:

> Call me jaded, but the fact that a retired radio technician, without a shred of medical background, is given credit for finding "a possible cure to cancer," when esteemed doctors and scientists have been shunned, imprisoned, and driven out of business for finding alternative cancer cures that actually work, is so preposterous you'd have to be born yesterday to believe there's no hidden agenda.

Indeed, this machine sounds remarkably similar to Raymond Rife's, whose treatment was proven to not harm surrounding healthy cells yet was rejected for conventional use. The hidden agenda that Dr Mercola refers to is the huge potential revenue this machine will generate for the cancer societies. Despite Kanzius developing the machine using his wife's pans, it would be a very expensive treatment when used conventionally. Nanoparticles are modern technology and it would be a dream come true for the scientific community to have it in all modern treatment facilities. Furthermore, the wholesale price of nanoparticles is $250 per 20 ml of nanoparticles[312] which means a guaranteed money-maker. Plus,

---

[312] http://www.nanocs.com/gold_nanoparticle.htm

wholesale prices are always the lowest possible; if the California books are anything to go by then a safe estimate would be a mark up of between seven to fifteen times the wholesale cost,[313] putting the price up to between $1,750 and $3,750 – for 20 ml.

In order for the safety of this machine to be tested adequately, a number of factors need to be considered. For example, are the radio-waves used at a similar frequency to those of healthy cells? Given that the purpose is to heat metal, the answer is probably negative, meaning there is a big possibility the healthy cells surrounding a tumour will be affected. John Kanzius putting his hand in the radio-wave field is not a reliable test as the frequency or duration could be too low to cause damage, but when both are increased for treatment purposes that could easily change. It must also be remembered that when Kanzius placed his hand in the radio-wave field he had no nanoparticles in his body, so he could not verify that there would be no side-effects. In fact, it is entirely possible that heating metal particles within the body could cause all manner of problems. There is also the problem of how the nanoparticles will be expelled from the body, as it would not be healthy or a wise idea to simply leave them there.

Whilst there is potential with this treatment, it certainly smacks more of chasing the money than a genuine, bonafide 'miracle cure' that it is being touted as. This is especially so given that Rife's safe, effective and cheap machine was rejected. In fact, all cheap, effective and safe therapies for cancer are rejected in favour of expensive, toxic and largely ineffective treatments. With the success rate of conventional cancer treatments being so low – lung cancer success is just 7%[314] – one would expect the institutes to be trying everything. With the proven and safe discoveries of Warburg and Budwig, they could be promoted at least in collaboration with chemotherapy and radiotherapy, but instead they are never mentioned. When one looks properly at the medical industry, the corruption and greed becomes instantly apparent, as the previous chapter highlighted.

Some people will be wondering what relevance any of this has to do with smoking or studies looking at the effects of smoking. Simply put, the cancer research institutes initiated much

---

[313] http://www.stopdown.net/med%20$%20Cal%20disclosure%20wsj.htm

[314] http://info.cancerresearchuk.org/cancerstats/types/lung/

of the war against smoking that we are currently suffering from and have intentionally neglected various forms of cancer treatment – opting instead to hinge success on drugs. They are also now organisations prompting specific ways of living rather than simply researching disease. Consequently, they are involved in the war against tobacco in a big way, and the rest of this chapter will be exploring this involvement.

The American Cancer Society (ACS)

The American Cancer Society has had some of the most powerful figures in banking, advertising and the entertainment industry on board, thus allowing them the advantage of changing policies. Elmer Holmes Bobst, a leading figure in the pharmaceutical industry and an Honorary Life Member of the ACS, wrote about the organisation in his 1973 autobiography. Entitled *Bobst: Autobiography of a Pharmaceutical Pioneer*, he states how it was initially a small affair and that he wanted to turn it into a much bigger machine:

> Governor Walte Edge, of New Jersey, and Eric Johnson, the czar of the motion picture industry, came to see me on behalf of the American Cancer society.... It had been run like a small mom and pop business, content to putter along with limited results... Without letting them know the reason, I invited all of my county bond chairmen and some other people of importance – about thirty in all – to join me for cocktails and dinner at a club...I explained, then, that I was about to undertake a mission...At the end of the evening, all but two of my bond volunteers, including nineteen of the county chairmen, agreed to join the crusade.

This excerpt highlights firstly the connections of the ACS, with Governor Walte Edge and Eric Johnson. It then explains how Bobst presented a slick evening to win over support for his campaign not to save lives, but to increase revenue:

> Within a few weeks...I was elected chairman of the executive committee...succeeding Emerson Foote, another great advertising leader...I decided that the first priority was

to **move aside the scientists and physicians** who were in administrative control of the organization. They were good men, but they were not experienced leaders, and **they were not getting results**. I wanted majority control to be in the hands of qualified lay leaders. The physician members could form a scientific committee to make recommendations about scientific matters and advise the executive committee [emphasis mine]

This excerpt could possibly be the most important in explaining the deceit and agenda rife within the ACS and other cancer research institutes. First and foremost, Bobst divulges another big name: Emerson Foote, an advertising leader. Next, and more importantly, he explains that the scientists and physicians were not producing the desired results so they were brushed aside and superseded by lay leaders instead. To put it in layman's terms, the real scientists were not producing results the ACS wanted to see, so instead they were removed from conducting the studies. Science was not top priority, propaganda and social control appeared to be instead.

Bobst admits in his book that he had a plan to change the structure of the ACS. In fact, prior to his taking over it was known as the American Society for the Control of Cancer (ASCC). The name change was more than aesthetic; it marked the turning point for when science no longer took precedence. To obtain full details of the restructuring, one must purchase the book – suffice it to say that such details are far too lengthy for this book. However, of notable importance to this topic is Bobst's plan to overcome the general public's ignorance of cancer. Though, of course, when one is ignorant, forthcoming information is accepted readily and passively – especially when originating from a seemingly respectable organisation such as the American Cancer Society. The so-called education plan began with the "Seven Danger Signals", which were: any sore that does not heal; a lump or thickening in the breast or elsewhere; unusual bleeding or discharge; any change in wart or mole; persistent indigestion or difficulty swallowing; persistent hoarseness or cough; any change in normal bowel habits.

Bobst is far from a man of modesty, and credits himself with bringing the attention of the ACS to Wynder and Graham's 1950 study that was reviewed in chapter five. He also credits himself with instigating the ACS's first epidemiological study. It was

Bobst's steering of the ACS that turned it into the anti-smoking machine it became:

> We released the first results of our study in June, 1954. Although the reactions of the tobacco industry, much of the public, and even many medical people ranged from outraged disbelief to quiet skepticism, we stuck by our guns and continued the study. As more reports came in and were evaluated, **we refined the results** to show that a person smoking one pack a day ran at least fourteen times more risk of lung cancer than the nonsmoker

A couple of things jump out of the text. Bobst admits they "refined" the results to show smoking elevates the risk of lung cancer. This is open to interpretation, but "refined" is not too far removed from 'changed'; and then one can wonder why they would refine the results if not to promote their own ideology. Also, the end of the quote has him saying that the evidence which has "conclusively put to rest" earlier denials is all based on his own research! To clarify, Bobst appeared to have the ACS undertake specific studies to prove his own point.

In 1945, Bobst was a member of the ACS Executive Committee, and Vice Chairman from 1946 to 1950. In 1947 to 1948 he was the ACS National Campaign Chairman and its chairman between 1949 and 1956. He became Honorary Board Chairman of the ACS in 1951 until 1955, and in 1956 to 1957 he was a director-at-large of the ACS.

Perhaps as the initial cause of things to come with the pharmaceutical companies, as highlighted in the previous chapter, Bobst was Chairman of the Board of Warner-Lambert Pharmaceutical Company; Director of the Spies Committee for Clinical Research; and a Trustee of Rutgers College of Pharmacy. He was also a member of the National Advisory Cancer Council of the National Cancer Institute. As a passing note, the patent for nicotine gum was held by Bobst's pharmaceutical company Warner-Lambert.

All in all, Bobst serves to highlight the corruption rampant in the cancer research organisations and their involvement in the anti-smoking crusade. Many of the studies linking smoking to lung cancer were funded by the ACS, a group run by Bobst who stated that he "refined" results and overcame scepticism by churning out studies based on his own findings. Most, if not all, of the early American smoking studies were created to appease the cancer research institutes, and the ACS was instrumental in producing those studies.

### The National Cancer Institute (NCI)

The National Cancer Institute is another respected and trusted organisation. The general public will trust an organisation with 'cancer' in the name, because it is a disease that affects us all; every person knows someone in their circle of family or friends who has suffered from cancer, whether it claimed their life or not. As such, we all want a cure and we trust those who set themselves up as officials. The NCI, though, like the ACS, has a public image that is merely a façade; behind the scenes things are very different. In fact, it is part of the federal government's National Institutes of Health.

In 2001, researcher Martha Perske wrote on the Forces website that she filed a Freedom of Information request, in 2000, to the National Cancer Institute asking for information on their funding Stanton Glantz's anti-smoking research.[315] They replied in 2001, just days before she posted on Forces, saying that the ongoing grant for Glantz's research is in its seventh year and will be ongoing until the twelfth year. They do not provide information of years one and two, but three to seven totals $2,074,576.00. Years eight to twelve, although not granted at the time of the response, were requested at $1,512,654.00. Although it was not granted then, we know now that Glantz did continue receiving money from the NCI and we are now eight years past that response. The total figure above is $3,587,230, or three million, five-hundred and eighty-seven thousand, two-hundred and thirty dollars. That is not including years one and two, or since the year 2006. So the actual number far exceeds that, but even three and a half million dollars is staggering.

As Perske rightly points out, cancer victims should be utterly appalled that a so-called cancer society is giving millions of dollars that could be well spent in various research centres to a fanatical anti-smoker – to conduct anti-smoking research! Cancer research societies should have no pre-set agenda. They are perfectly entitled to conduct research into smoking, but objectively. Authorising biased studies with a pre-determined outcome is

---

[315] http://www.forces.org/research/files/nci.htm

unscientific and failing millions of people worldwide. Moreover, the NCI, and indeed the ACS, fund Glantz's political work. Below is a repeat of Glantz's quote from chapter six:

> In each state one or two politicians seem to be taking the lead in pushing the industry's position (at least publicly). As soon as these politicians start floating trial balloons, they should be attacked publicly. If they can be bloodied, it could well scare the others off. Fear is a great motivator for politicians.[316]

Glantz is not an objective researcher by any stretch of the imagination. Furthermore, his past and his openness about his disdain of smokers leave no doubt that the NCI know exactly who they are funding, and what they are funding him for. This is stark evidence that the cancer research institutes are promoting anti-smoking junk science for their own gain.

The July 1995 issue of *Alternative in Philanthropy* talks about the NCI and how it has provided anti-smoking organisations with as much as $100 million in federal tax revenues, for the sole purpose of lobbying for higher tobacco taxes. Put another way, a cancer research institution has provided a tenth of a billion dollars to just one small part of the anti-smoking crusade. That makes Glantz's research grant look like a drop in the ocean. All the while, the NCI is asking the public for generous donations so they can help beat cancer. It truly beggars belief. The major funding for this comes from the NCI's Project ASSIST, which stands for the American Stop Smoking Intervention Study for Cancer Prevention. Note how the acronym ends with the 't' in 'study', rather than being ASSISCP – to appear as though they are 'assisting' smokers.

According to the article, Project ASSIST was spearheaded mostly by the ACS and it supports grassroots groups that organise campaigns which 'educate' the public in an attempt to discourage smoking. The article itself is a follow-up which examines the operation of ASSIST in Colorado, showing how federal funds were illegally used to try to raise the state's tobacco tax. The full article

---

[316] www.smokescreen.org

can be viewed online,[317] and is reported on the Forces website.[318] The article begins thusly:

> Dr. James T Bennett, a professor of economics at George Mason University in Fairfax, Virginia, has criticized the ACS for spending too little on direct services for cancer victims while conducting unnecessary public education programs, funding seminars for well-to-do medical professionals, and amassing real estate .
>
> In the two articles in this issue, Bennett discusses how some ACS affiliates have been less than forthcoming in providing information about their spending practices and how the ACS is increasingly embroiled in politics.

Dr James Bennett wrote:

> What emerges is a complex and twisted tale: front groups were created to provide a smokescreen for lobbying; state bureaucrats used state offices to facilitate lobbying; and positions of authority were sold, with those hoping to acquire a share of the projected tax revenue paying "front money" to secure positions.

Anti-smoking groups had been active for over a decade when Project ASSIST came to fruition, and one of their primary goals was to raise taxes on tobacco products. The constitution of Colorado permits citizen-initiated referenda, thus making Colorado perfect for Project ASSIST to pursue this agenda. The National Cancer Institute gave the Colorado Department of Health (CDH) a contract which provided them almost $7 million dollars ($6,976,683 to be exact) between the 20th September 1991 and the 29th September 1998, almost $1 million annually. In turn, the CDH provided funds from Project ASSIST to local anti-smoking groups. To put this into perspective: the NCI, a government health institute, provided a state with seven million dollars over a seven year period in return for the ability to aid anti-smoking groups. The motive is

---

[317]http://legacy.library.ucsf.edu/tid/kaf97d00/ pdf;jsessionid=FB67E8FA54836479A87A3F8E5441B655

[318] http://www.forces.org/evidence/assist/bennett1.htm

clear: grassroots organisations typically carry more weight with the public as it then appears to be a movement of genuine concern rather than a corporate movement. The latter run the risk of public rejection as corporations or the government removing their rights. Thus, by controlling local groups the NCI furthered their agenda.

Thanks to Colorado permitting citizen-initiated referenda, anti-smoking activists filed an "initiative regarding Tobacco Taxes" with the Colorado Department of State on the 19th November 1993. If the initiative passed, taxes would be raised on July 1st 1995 by fifty cents per pack for cigarettes, and cigars and smokeless tobacco products being increased by 50% of the manufacturer's list price. The aim, apparently, was to cut smoking rates by 43% in Colorado, but it appears this was not the case – if it were, higher taxes would have been sufficient. However, an estimated $130 million per year in tax revenues were to be distributed in the following way:

- $65 million to medical professionals and hospitals for health care of the needy;

- $39 million to anti-smoking activists and health charities for educational programs to reduce tobacco use;

- $13 million to academics and public interest groups for research on tobacco use.

Further to this, $13 million was to be split among counties, municipalities, economic development initiatives and an eleven-member citizens' commission. The eleven members would oversee the disbursement of revenues and would most probably be health charity officials, medical professionals, and anti-smoking activists. This can be seen by the table in appendix three, showing that the Fair Share for Health Committee (FSFHC), a lobbying organisation created to promote the tax initiative, consisted of Colorado hospital, medical and health charity professions. Colorado ASSIST, an educational organisation set-up to receive Project ASSIST funds, has a noticeable membership overlap with the FSFHC. Furthermore, the Colorado ASSIST's executive committee included representatives of the ACS, Colorado Department of Health, and the Coalition for a Tobacco-Free Colorado (CTFC). To break this information down once more, a federal government organisation paid substantial sums specifically to lobby the Colorado state for increased tobacco taxes.

The National Cancer Institute was aware that Colorado ASSIST's aim was to raise state taxes. They were also aware that federal funds would be used to push the initiative. The Colorado Department of Health submitted documents to the NCI that repeatedly emphasised the tax theme:

- Colorado should "increase economic incentives and taxation to discourage the use of tobacco products;"

- "The price of tobacco products needs to be greatly increased through taxes and/or sales-license fees;"

- "The Colorado ASSIST Alliance will work to increase public knowledge of the need to increase the cigarette tax substantially;"

- "Educational presentations will be made to all [areas] regarding the need and current efforts to increase tobacco taxes;"

- "Strategies to advocate increased tobacco taxes will be incorporated into the ASSIST media plan;"

- "Information will be presented...regarding the rationale and need for sales license fees on tobacco sales."

Further to this, the Colorado Department of Health had other materials which clearly showed that ASSIST funds were being used for political activity. ASSIST consultant and founding board member of the CTFC Connie Acott submitted expense reports to the CDH which note that the Colorado ASSIST meetings concerning the "tax initiative" and the "coalition tax initiative" were held in August and November of 1992. Another Colorado ASSIST expense report highlights a meeting of the organisation's "Political Advocacy Team" on April 15th 1993.

In addition to the above, ASSIST funded many organisations that were promoting the tobacco tax hike. Appendix four of this book contains a table showing just a partial list of groups that received ASSIST contracts between 1993 and 1994, and comparing that table to the one in Appendix three shows that a lot of money was given to organisations that were part of the Fair Share For Health tax initiative.

Not only were the funds provided, but recipients were required to fill out contract reimbursement forms and an "Activity Matrix". One of the goals of the Activity Matrix was "Economic

Incentive to Decrease Tobacco Use" in the following ways: "educate re excise taxes", "attend training", and "coordinate publicity/media". Let us not forget that all the money given to these organisations came directly from tax-payers – meaning that, in short, smokers and non-smokers were paying the government so they could create dictatorial and manipulative groups to tell the public how to live. It seems that the ACS and NCI forgot that their role should be to research causes and treatments for a disease, not to give away vast sums of money to health groups. Lifestyle control is not the job of cancer research institutes. As Dr. Bennett wrote towards the end of the aforementioned article:

> The ACS should return to its traditional mission of providing direct services to cancer patients – a mission it has increasingly abandoned in favor of lobbying for restrictions on personal behavior.

Quite right. And so, too, should the NCI.


Cancer Research UK


Cancer Research UK (CRUK) is another cancer research institution; although unlike the ACS and NCI it does receive most of its funding from donations. Like the ACS and NCI, however, it is not so much a genuine charity to improve public health but rather an organisation that tries to change the lifestyle choices of the public. Rather than do this through education, it chooses to fund research that will force people to change their lifestyles through fear. Of course, it will not admit such propaganda; in fact, their website states in big, bold letters "our research saves lives".[319] Perhaps somebody should explain to them that the fear they instil in people is actually more likely to lead to the onset of disease and, consequently, death.

Cancer Research UK is a staunch anti-smoking group; it even has its own Tobacco Advisory Group (TAG) which:

> was established to oversee the charity's tobacco policies and tobacco policy research. Cancer Research UK provides major/significant funding towards several important

---

[319] http://science.cancerresearchuk.org/

tobacco control organisations. This funding is overseen by the TAG.[320]

We are also told that TAG:

> particularly funds research and activities that support:
> * Smokefree workplaces across the UK and internationally, and other measures to protect against second-hand smoke exposure;
> * Greater regulation of all tobacco and nicotine-containing products;
> * Development and implementation of the WHO treaty, the 'Framework Convention on Tobacco Control';
> * Greater tax/smuggling measures in the UK and internationally;
> * UK tobacco research needs; building research capacity and supporting research in to practice;
> * Tacking health inequalities and addressing the needs of groups with particularly high rates of tobacco use.

This shows very clearly that CRUK is not interested in objective research of tobacco smoking, but only in anti-smoking. Note how it does not say TAG funds studies looking into smoking effects, but only studies showing it is harmful. To prove the point further, CRUK provides examples of studies and areas it has funded. One notable example is that it part-funds Action on Smoking and Health (ASH), a group dedicated to continually penalising smokers. ASH receives money from the Department of Health and ASH International, which is part-funded by pharmaceutical giant Pfizer. A second example is that it funds the Centre for Tobacco Control Research (CTCR), University of Stirling. According to CRUK:

> The Centre develops and evaluates interventions designed to prevent smoking uptake and encourage cessation; investigates the processes and effects of the tobacco

---

[320] http://science.cancerresearchuk.org/gapp/fundingcommittees/

industry's marketing activities and evaluates specific tobacco control policies to identify those that successfully change smoking behaviour.[321]

Cancer Research UK does not merely fund UK or European initiatives. It also funds internationally and, along with the ACS and CTCR, funds "various grants schemes for advocates in low- and middle-income countries."[322] Again with the ACS, CRUK funds the African Tobacco Control Resource Initiative, which helps support information and capacity building in sub-Saharan Africa. Cancer Research UK also funds the Global Smokefree Partnership, which, as the name suggests, "aims to promote effective smokefree air policies worldwide."[323] The last example on the TAG webpage is "research to examine appropriate stop smoking services in parts of China."

As we can clearly see, Cancer Research UK is working very hard to demonise and limit smoking around the world, not just in Britain. A global campaign is underway, and the biggest cancer research institutions play a big part. Interestingly, Cancer Research UK, a supposed charity, is a limited company[324].

The fruits of their labours, and further recognition of their agenda, can be seen by a cursory glance at their page on cancer. They have a drop-down list of twenty-six types of cancer, but where they list lung cancer rather than merely saying the name, they say "lung cancer and smoking."[325] The only cause of lung cancer that it mentions is smoking. They do acknowledge radon as a factor, saying "radon is a naturally occurring gas that increases risk of lung cancer, especially among smokers."[326] So, even when they acknowledge that there is another factor in the onset of lung

---

[321] http://science.cancerresearchuk.org/gapp/fundingcommittees/tag/

[322] Ibid.

[323] Ibid.

[324] http://www.cancerresearchuk.org/

[325] http://info.cancerresearchuk.org/cancerstats/types/lung/

[326] Ibid

cancer, they still have to state that smokers are more likely to suffer. There is not a shred of objective research on the whole page.

They notice a large discrepancy that the countries with the highest rates of smoking have lower rates of lung cancer, but they say "this will change if the current trends in the uptake of smoking persist in countries like China." Evidently they are unaware that these countries have been smoking heavily for a long time, as shown in both Wynder's study in chapter five and the sub-chapter "World Data". Another highly relevant point is that they admit 75% of people diagnosed with lung cancer are aged sixty-five or over; thus proving once more that cancer is predominately a disease of the elderly. Despite this, though, they still tell people that smoking will lead to premature death.

They also admit that the survival rates of lung cancer are only 7%. Perhaps this is an indication that they should stop deliberately lying to the public and should focus instead on what they are supposed to be doing – objectively researching ways to cure cancer.

Oddly enough, this information is on the lung cancer fact page for health professionals; they have a separate page for the public. For some reason the information is slightly different on the two pages, with the public one acknowledging there are other risks but also taking pains to emphasise that they are not as important or dangerous as smoking: "Some other things increase lung cancer risk, but they increase the risk far less than smoking"[327]

They also make the error in insinuating that correlation equals causation, by saying "Although some people who have never smoked get lung cancer, smoking causes 9 out of 10 cases." Really and truly, all that they can say is lung cancer occurs 90% of the time in smokers but, for the reasons I have shown throughout the course of this book, that is not reason to believe it is *because* of smoking. Furthermore, they ignore the fact that most smokers do not get the disease. Their own figures show it is a rare disease: they state there are eleven million smokers in the United Kingdom, and that 38,598 are diagnosed with lung cancer each year. This means that 0.3% of smokers contract lung cancer a year, hardly the gigantic figure they speak of routinely. The eleven million they use is also a conservative figure as it does not account for those who buy abroad or from the

---

[327] http://www.cancerhelp.org.uk/help/default.asp?page=2962

black market. In reality, the number could be nearer to twelve million.

In truth, if the cancer organisations truly were about helping people then the main focus would not be tobacco. Even if we accept that smoking is the main cause of lung cancer that still leaves numerous other cancers and countless possible causes. The cancer research institutions have played a huge part in the anti-smoking movements that we are seeing the world over. Cancer Research UK even openly admits such involvement on its website; such is the public opinion now that such 'research' is well-meaning and justified. In truth, it is neither. It is manipulation and public control. Such organisations should not be involved in changing the public's lifestyles, but should be conducting objective research and providing the information to the public for them to make their own minds up. As Thomas Jefferson said in 1775: "False is the idea...that would take fire from men because it burns and water because one may drown in it; that has no remedy for evils, except destruction [of liberty]".[328]

---

[328]http://legacy.library.ucsf.edu/tid/kaf97d00/ pdf;jsessionid=FB67E8FA54836479A87A3F8E5441B655 p.7

## Summation

This book has examined in detail the evidence that is used to convince the public that smoking is harmful. In the process it has shown that the evidence is not only unconvincing but that it fails to prove a link between smoking and any illness or disease, let alone making it accountable for millions of deaths. The anti-smoking movement has been shown to be largely an initial product of intolerant individuals wanting their own way, and later taken under the wings of cancer research institutions and the pharmaceutical industry. The latter saw a very profitable target in the smoker wanting to give up out of fear, expense or consciously engineered social pressure.

A lot of people say they believe smoking kills because they know someone who died as a result of smoking. This is not proof, it is anecdotal. After all, doctors and researchers still do not know *how* smoking causes cancer or any other disease attributed to it, so all they have to go on is a statistical link. However, a chief problem with this is that lots of other factors are ignored, and studies typically just look at how many cigarettes are smoked and then say smoking kills. As Aaron Levenstein famously stated: "Statistics are like bikinis. What they reveal is suggestive, but what they conceal is vital." Furthermore, statistical link is not much better than pure assumption; for instance, if a handful of fifty-five year-old smokers who died of a heart attack were collated then a statistical link could be generated, even though many non-smoking fifty-five year olds also die of heart attacks.

The truth is that people have been smoking tobacco for quite literally thousands of years. Given this, smoking is perhaps one of the oldest pastimes of pleasure and if it really were as deadly as we are to believe then the population would not be nearly as large as it is. People point out that we have only realised how dangerous smoking is through the advancements of medicine and science. However, this fails to stand up to scrutiny because we know that tobacco has been smoked widely for thousands of years, yet the population has never suffered for it. We also have the luxury of being able to see very different smoking trends and patterns from the past seventy years and seeing that they appear to have had no effect on life expectancy or population rates.

Despite all the attention that smoking receives for causing lung cancer and heart disease, there is not an epidemic of either. In fact, even though smokers are statistically more likely to get lung cancer than non-smokers, the increase is very small and only 10-15% of smokers actually contract cancer. With all the hyperbole and attention given to smoking causing this disease and that disease, and 50% of smokers apparently dying from the habit, the truth has been blown out of all proportion. That truth is simple: there is no evidence that smoking is harmful.

There is, though, lots of evidence that smoking is beneficial. No animal study has ever succeeded in producing lung cancer with tobacco, even more recently where F334 rats and A/J mice, specially bred to develop cancers, have been used, the smoke-exposed ones outlived the animals living in smokefree conditions. Human studies have been manipulated to produce the desired results, but no study that has been released with the raw data has supported the hypothesis that smoking is a deadly habit. Many researchers and physicians have spoken out against the claim that smoking causes disease. Furthermore, the rates of smoking have been declining since the 1960s and only recently have reached a plateau, yet the incidence of diseases linked to smoking, such as emphysema and lung cancer, has risen with tremendous speed.

This book has shown how detection bias is a very real problem, leading to bogus statistics and misrepresentative figures. Sadly, these figures and statistics are used in the mainstream media, thus leading people to believe smoking is a deadly habit. The book has also shown how social class plays a very big role in disease, because lifestyles vary greatly between people of different social statuses. Statistically, most smokers are from the lower classes and, accordingly, they tend to suffer more illness – not just cancer, but depression, stress and others, and even a statistically increased likelihood of committing suicide. As Dr Denson so aptly stated, we must not confuse smoker-related illness with smoking-related illness.

Why do smokers get more disease? There are numerous reasons why smokers appear to suffer from higher incidence of disease, from a physical perspective. This includes such 'physicality's' as detection bias and social class. There is, however, another suggestion: Western medicine has thoroughly overlooked the metaphysical state of existence i.e. the effect of the brain or mind on the body and its overall wellbeing. To quote Dr Ian Dunbar, who wrote the foreword to this book:

The mind is a source of widespread biochemical changes affecting the whole body. For example if an individual feels insecure for any reason the mind experiences anxiety. This is associated with adrenaline, a hormone that has widespread effects not only on the mind but on the heart, lungs, brain, central nervous system, muscles, gut and blood. Excluding the mind from scientific research has therefore excluded consideration of the part played by powerful variables such as adrenaline.

Putting this in perspective of the smoking debate, it is a well known fact that many smokers use the habit to relieve stress or calm their nerves. One aspect science has overlooked is *why* people smoke: there are those who started smoking through peer pressure or curiousity and continued through habit or enjoyment, and there are those who smoke as a means of 'self-medication' – to help them cope with the pressures of everyday life.

Research tells us that stress and an unbalanced mind can cause heart disease and cancer. The latter group of the types of smokers mentioned above are instantly at increased risk of both types of illness for the simple fact of being stressed or otherwise 'unbalanced'. Thus, the statistical link shows smoking being related to heart disease or cancer, whereas in actual fact the smoking signifies another link: that of the mind, or stress. Science has spent over half a century attempting to prove smoking causes lung cancer and other ailments, but all it has ever achieved is a statistical link. Statistically, birthdays appear good for us because those who have the most of them live longest – yet we know it is not the birthday itself that leads to longevity, they merely mark the amount of time a person has existed. In short: a statistical link between smoking and disease is not proof of a causal link. A causal link cannot be shown until all areas are thoroughly covered, and all the while reasons behind the choice to smoke or the mental and physical state of the smoker are ignored there are serious areas lacking in research.

Right now history is repeating itself; we have seen prohibition with alcohol and we have seen many attacks on smoking. The continuous onslaught against tobacco reveals the façade that the issue is one that is political in nature, not scientific. If it truly were the latter then the science would be objective and not the result of anti-smoking groups such as Cancer Research's subsidiary TAG. One example is how we are told that pure,

269

additive-free tobacco is no safer than mass produced cigarettes, despite there being no study or evidence to test if this is true.

If history is anything to go by, then the probability is that this war will end in the foreseeable future and people can smoke in luxury again, but that does not mean people should not learn the truth to stop it happening again and to help this one end a little earlier. Despite history teaching us the lesson, we still insist on letting intolerant megalomaniacs hold all the power which they use to demonise the masses. For once, it is time the masses rose up to ensure equality. The loudest and strongest voice is not democracy, nor is eradicating the minority. Whilst it may be true that smokers are the minority, they are a large minority and deserve as much consideration and thought as non-smokers, such is the beauty of living in a democratic nation.

This book will finish with two things. First is an interesting timeline of tobacco, for the reader to view online, which shows how it was first used, what it was used for, such as cures and treatments, and past attacks on smokers.[329] Second are some quotes from doctors and medical practitioners; these quotes first appeared in *The Smoking Scare De-Bunked* by Dr Whitby.[330]

Professor Burch, University of Leeds: "Smoking has no role in lung cancer."

Dr R.H. Mole, British Medical Research Council: "Evidence in uranium miners permits the exclusion of smoking as a major causal agent."

Dr B.K.S. Dijkstra, University of Pretoria: "The natural experi-ment shows conclusively that the hypothesis has to be abandoned."

Professor Sir Ronald Fisher, late of Cambridge University: "The theory will eventually be regarded as a catastrophic and conspicuous howler."

Dr Ronald Okun, Director of Clinical Pathology, Los Angeles: "As a scientist I find no persuasive evidence that cigarette smoke causes lung cancer."

---

[329]http://communities.canada.com/ottawacitizen/blogs/quittingtime/archive/
2008/03/04/cleaning-the-superfluous-humours-of-the-brain-and-the-
accompanying-withering-of-the-noble-parts.aspx

[330] http://legacy.library.ucsf.edu/cgi/getdoc?
tid=isfl4d00&fmt=pdf&ref=results

Professor W.C . Hueper, National Cancer Institute, Switzerland: "Scientifically unsound and socially irresponsible."

Professor M:B. Rosenblatt, New York Medical College, "It is fanciful extrapolation – not factual data."

Professor Sheldon Sommers, New York Academy of Medicine and Science: "The belief that smoking is the cause of lung cancer is no longer widely held by scientists," and also, "Smoking is no longer seen as a cause of heart disease except by a few zealots."

# Appendix 1

## Why?

If the use of tobacco is not injurious,
WHY does the life insurance company wish to know whether the applicant smokes?
WHY does the surgeon, contemplating a serious operation, ask whether the patient smokes?
WHY are athletes, in training, forbidden to smoke?

## Efficiency Destroyers

BOYS know that rum and whisky are efficiency destroyers. They look with disgust or pity upon the drunkard, the man who has voluntarily destroyed his efficiency by drinking liquor. But the boy who smokes is walking in the same path that the drunkard took. To the growing boy the cigarette is as great an evil as rum is to the man. When the man takes his first drink, and the boy smokes his first cigarette, the two start on the efficiency - destroying path; for as the first glass of whisky usually in time leads to the gutter, so the first cigarette usually leads to the inefficiency and debility of the cigarette fiend. A cigarette-smoking boy is a fifty-per-cent loss to every good cause. It has been scientifically proved that smoking produces grave effects on mind, body, and soul. Dr. A. E. Gilson, of the United States Navy, cites the following list of evils resulting from the habitual use of the harmful weed:

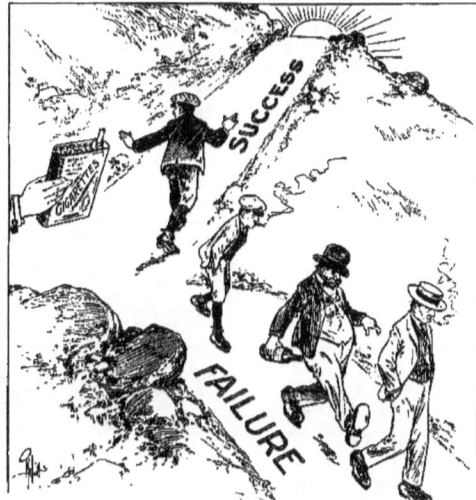

"'It leads to impaired nutrition of the nerve centers.
"'It is a fertile cause of neuralgia, vertigo, and indigestion.
"'It irritates the mouth and throat, and thus destroys the purity of the voice.
"'By excitation of the optic nerves it provokes amaurosis and other defects of vision.
"'It causes a tremulous hand and an intermittent pulse.
"'One of its conspicuous effects is to develop irritability of the heart.
"'It retards the cell change upon which the development of the adolescent depends.'
"It will be remembered that when the Boer War broke out, 11,000 volunteered for service in the Manchester District alone; 8,000 of whom were at once rejected as physically unfit, and only 1,200 finally passed the doctors. The chief cause of unfitness was proved to be smoking by boys and young men."

To the sensible boy the strongest testimony against the cigarette is the fact that so many of life's business doors are closed to cigarette users.

### Signing the Pledge

HELLO, Walter! what is that you find so interesting that you nearly stumble over a fellow?"
"An anti-cigarette pledge Tom Brown just handed me. Perhaps you've seen it."
"Yes, indeed; James and I both signed it long ago; and of course you intend to."
"Not much. It is unmanly. Only weak men sign pledges."
"So you call a pledge unmanly?"
"Certainly, and hundreds of men say the same thing."
"If you won't sign a pledge, you will have to go to some desert island and live all by yourself, for in our country the pledge is the basis of social and business life. You can never witness in a legal suit."
"If my testimony was needed to aid right and secure justice, I should be willing to serve as a witness."
"But you would have to pledge yourself to tell nothing but the truth. I suppose that would be unmanly."
"No, that is different."

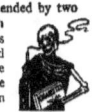

true manliness demands the refusal. We are free from the idea "that honor can in any way be mended by two men standing up to take snapshots at each other." But we have been freed from this superstitious idea because some men had enough true courage and manliness to dare to be thought unmanly and cowardly by the majority, holding the narrower and mistaken

"If you go into business, you will have to be unmanly enough to sign a good many pledges, or you cannot lease a house, sign a note or any kind of contract, for they are all pledges. And you cannot be President of the United States, for you would have to take the pledge of office. And you cannot get married when you grow up, for then you would have to take a pledge."
"I guess you have the best of it, James. I never thought of it in this light before. But an anti-cigarette pledge is a different thing. I don't smoke and never intend to. I don't need to sign any pledge."
"How about your influence over the fellows who do need it? If we are free from evil, we set a good example for the smaller boys; and if we sign the pledge, it is easier for others to do so. That's right, Walter."
"I suppose that is true," admitted Walter.
"Of course it is. Come and help us along," urged both boys of their comrade. "All right. Where's a pencil?"— *Adapted from Boys' Companion.*

### Do It

If you have any interest in the American boy, do something at once to save him from the cigarette habit. In lots of fifty or more this paper can be had for 4 cents a copy. Will you not place it in the hands of at least fifty boys?

JUDGE LINDSEY says: "I know of no habit more responsible for the troubles of boys than the vile cigarette habit. No pure-minded, honest, manly boy will smoke cigarettes."

## The Youth's Instructor

ISSUED TUESDAYS BY THE

### REVIEW AND HERALD PUBLISHING ASSN.

TAKOMA PARK STATION, WASHINGTON, D. C.

FANNIE DICKERSON CHASE - - - - - *Editor*
ADELAIDE BEE EVANS - - - - *Associate Editor*

| LXV | AUGUST 28, 1917 | No. 35 |
|---|---|---|

Entered as second-class matter, August 14, 1903, at the post office, at Washington, D. C., under the act of Congress of March 3, 1879.

# The Youth's Instructor

TAKOMA PARK STATION · ANTI-TOBACCO ANNUAL · WASHINGTON, D. C.

## When a Boy Knows More Than His Father

SOMETIMES a boy *does* know more than his father. Ours would have been a very different history if Abe Lincoln, age sixteen or so, had been guided by the wisdom of Thomas Lincoln, age thirty-six or so.

"Now, Abe," we can imagine him saying, "don't waste time readin' them books. Readin' never done me any good, and what was good enough for me's good enough for you."

Lincoln knew more than his father. It was a divine disobedience that led him to close his ears to the man who had brought him into the world, and open his heart to the vision that was to help him conquer the world.

Robert Louis Stevenson knew more than his father. That father would have shackled him to the dry problems of engineering. He

His path looked golden and long. And then suddenly he stopped.

"You see that man?" said the president of his concern to me the other day. "There is a man who might have become general manager of this concern if he had had a college education. His salary might have been $20,000 a year; instead it's $2,000. He's reached his limit. What a shame that he hasn't education enough to go on."

He "knew more" than his father. And his boyish obstinacy is costing him $18,000 a year.

I know another man who "knew more" than his father. "Keep yourself clean, my son," said the father to him. "You'll never regret it. And some day you'll be glad you did." But the boy knew more than his father. He knew that every young

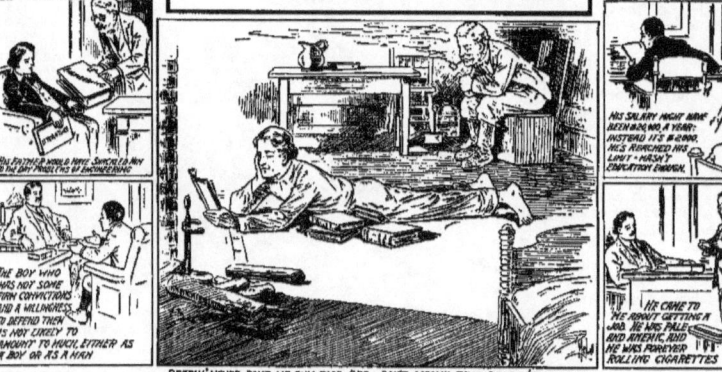

*READIN' NEVER DONE ME ANY GOOD, ABE. DON'T WASTE TIME READIN' THEM BOOKS.*

could not understand the obstinacy of the boy who refused to apply himself. That obstinacy saved a great author from misery as a mediocre engineer. That obstinacy enriched the ages.

"Let no man despise thy youth," wrote Paul to Timothy.

The boy who has not some firm convictions and a willingness to defend them, even against the arguments of those older than himself, is not likely to amount to much either as a boy or as a man.

But they must be *convictions*, not mere *prejudices*, not *selfish impulses or passions*.

I know two men who "knew more" than their fathers. One boy is the office manager of a large manufacturing concern, and his salary is $40 a week.

"Better go on in school," said his father to him when he was seventeen years old. "Better go to college; better get all the education you can while you have the chance. You'll need it afterward."

But the boy quit school and went to work.

He was promoted from office boy to bookkeeper, from bookkeeper to head bookkeeper, from head bookkeeper to office manager.

man must sow his wild oats. So he sowed right merrily.

I saw him the other day. He came to me about getting a job.

He was pale, and anemic, and his hands twitched, and he was forever rolling cigarettes. He could not concentrate his mind on one subject for even two minutes.

I couldn't give him a job: no man could. God knows what will become of him. He would starve if it were not for the few dollars he gets from his father—

The father who, he thought, didn't know so much as he. — *Bruce Barton, Editor, in Every Week.*

### What a $1,200,000,000 Tobacco Investment Brings the Smokers

THE Postal Life Insurance Company of New York City, having large opportunities of observation, in speaking of the effect of tobacco upon adults, says:

"Tobacco covers nearly the whole range of human ills, dyspepsia, catarrhal troubles of the nose and throat, heart disturbances, nervous irritability, trembling, and impaired eyesight."

(*Concluded on page sixteen*)

273

### Luther Burbank, the Plant Wizard

MR. BURBANK is to the plant world what Mr. Edison is to the electric world. His wand can give to the calla lily the fragrance of violets or of water lilies, and to the plum the fragrance and flavor of the Bartlett pear. Seedless oranges, stoneless plums, white blackberries, and a long list of new varieties of fruits and flowers are products of his wizardry. Out of a black walnut tree and a California walnut he has produced a new tree that grows twice as rapidly as the combined growth of both parents. The ordinary chestnut tree of the woods requires from ten to fifteen years to pass from seedling stage to nut bearing; but Mr. Burbank has made a chestnut tree six months old bear nuts. The pineapple quince, a luscious fruit, which combines the characteristic qualities of each of the parents; the Burbank potato, known throughout the country; and the spineless cactus, which because of its economic

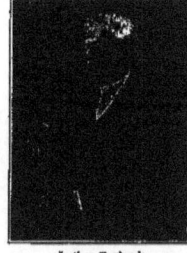

*Luther Burbank*

value is regarded by some as his greatest achievement, are all products of Mr. Burbank's skill. He has produced the Australian star flower, which retains permanently its perfume and color; the scarlet poppy, yellow calla lily, new and hardy varieties of the tea rose; and besides these he has combined the field daisy with Japanese and European varieties, producing the exquisite Shasta daisy, a prince among flowers. All this has Mr. Burbank done, and much more. But there is one thing he has not done. I have asked him to tell you himself. He says:

"I have never used tobacco in any form, and, being of a nervous temperament, I am entirely satisfied that I should not have survived if I had. Many of my young friends are now in their graves, undoubtedly from cigarette smoking alone. I have never met any person who thought that cigarettes were beneficial to any one, under any circumstances. Why do people use them? That is too much for me, for the effect of them on boys is exactly like that of sand in a watch."

Mr. Burbank absolutely refuses to employ cigarette users in his gardens, for he says that tobacco destroys the delicacy of touch necessary in his budding work. So our wonder-working plant wizard of America says, both by example and precept, that boys who wish to do things worth while must not touch the filthy weed, tobacco.

---

### What a $1,200,000,000 Tobacco Investment Brings the Smokers
*(Concluded from page one)*

The Life Extension Institute says:

"Tobacco used freely causes inflammation of the throat, and invites the attack of germs."

Phipps Institute showed by a series of observations that smokers are twice as likely to have tuberculosis as non-smokers.

The founders of the Spencerian Business College, after thirty years of observation of young people, say:

"The effects of this narcotic are premature age, shattered nerves, mental weakness, stunted growth, and general physical and moral degeneracy; and therefore we decline to receive into our institution any who use this noxious weed."

It is very rare for a smoker to take high honors in his class. In some colleges such a thing has not happened in fifty years, although the smokers are many and the abstainers few.

Nine tenths of army rejections are said to be due to tobacco heart. It has been proved that the excessive use of tobacco —

| | |
|---|---|
| Checks growth | Seriously interferes with circulation and respiration |
| Causes tobacco heart | |
| Promotes cancers | Weakens morals |
| Injures eyesight, frequently causing blindness | Excludes religion |
| | Offends society |
| Impairs intellect | Makes criminals |
| Lowers scholarship | Lessens business efficiency |
| Injures nerves | Unfits for athletic sports |
| Destroys sensitiveness of taste | Creates craving oftentimes for liquor |
| Predisposes to tuberculosis | |
| Impairs work of kidneys | Poisons family |

Not all tobacco users suffer from all of these afflictions, yet one may be assured that if the use of tobacco is begun early in youth and continued to manhood, the majority of these ills will manifest themselves. To a regular but moderate user who did not begin until years of manhood were reached, the ill effects are not so grave, but any one of the most serious results is likely to manifest itself in an unexpected moment, and demand the death toll.

---

### Undeceive the Boys

ARE the boys altogether to be censured for considering smoking as an element of manliness, when ever movie hero sports a cigar or cigarette; when nearly a clothing illustrations show boys or men smoking; whe high-class magazine illustrations represent the hero of the story with his cigar; when great advertising billboard show the men with pipe, cigar, or cigarette; when the daily newspapers devote whole pages to advertising matter setting forth the pleasure of the smoking habit; and when every street car has one or more signs telling of the delights of some kind of tobacco?

All this is but part of a nation-wide campaign to catch the boys as cigarette buyers, that the coffers of the American Tobacco Company may overflow with dollars from the destruction of the souls and bodies of our boys.

A duel is to be fought. The great tobacco trust is on one side, the great army of American boys on the other One of these will succumb. Which it shall be depend upon you and me, and all the rest of those who love an believe in the boys.

It is evident that boys will be misled by the strenuous effort on the part of the tobacco trust to make them thin that smoking and manliness go together. It is our part to undeceive them, and let them know that the higher manhood is divorced from the tobacco evil. It is for me to show them by total abstinence that true manhood eschews the weed. When will men sense the responsibility

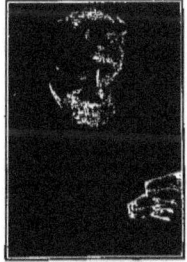

that rests upon them in th fight to free the boys from the cigarette curse? Right example is better for boy than sermons.

---

### An Inventor's Word

HUDSON MAXIM, the inventor of the mult perforated smokeless powder grain; inventor of maximit the first high explosive to be fired from a cannon with powder through armor plate the inventor of motorite, material which by self-combustion drives the torped

*Copyright by Harris & Ewing*
*Hudson Maxim*

through the water at from forty-five to sixty miles an hour; and of many other important inventions, speaks in no undertone about the evil effect of tobacco when he says: "Tobacco is a maker of invalids, criminals, an fools!" His latest word on the subject comes as a personal word to the readers of this issue. He says:

"No, I do not smoke. Tobacco is one of the greatest evils of the modern world. It is one of the great degenerators of the race.

"None of my direct ancestry, as far back as I am able to trace ever used tobacco, consequently tobacco is unusually poisonous to me through lack of immunity. Up to the time I was thirty-five years old I found the use of tobacco by others an insufferable nuisance. Frequently I would become so poisoned by tobacco smoke as to be ill for days. One time in London while attending a dinner I was made sick for six weeks."

# A Physician's Advice to Boys

D. H. KRESS, M. D.

LOOK before you jump, boys. Before smoking the first cigarette, ascertain where it may land you. I know where it has landed some boys. I have seen the prospects of many a boy ruined by the cigarette. Promising boys by the hundred have made a failure of life because they took the first smoke.

The cigarette habit, when taken up by boys before the brain is fully developed, brings about a degeneracy of the brain cells, and may produce a moral insanity. It tends to develop criminal tendencies.

Ninety-eight per cent of the inmates of the Whittier Reform School in California are cigarette smokers. All cigarette smokers do not become criminals, but practically all youthful criminals are cigarette smokers. These facts are known to judges of all our juvenile courts. It is practically certain that the boy who lands in the police court smokes; and it is equally certain that many a boy would never have been there if he had not smoked.

I said to a Chicago detective during the time when the city was being terrorized by youthful automobile bandits, "Haven't you found that in nearly every case these young criminals are cigarette fiends?" He looked at me a moment, and then replied, "In every case." One of these cases, Teddy Webb, who was then arrested and is now serving a life sentence for murdering a policeman, was a fine, promising boy at the age of ten years. At that age he began to use cigarettes with the boys in the alleys. His downward career began at that point. At the age of eleven he robbed an old woman on the street, and began to figure in the police court. His downward career continued until he reached his present low estate.

The boy who has an ambition to excel in life, whose aim is to climb to the top, cannot afford to take chances. He will leave cigarettes alone. The cigarette has never yet placed a boy in the chair of the President of this nation. Lincoln was a poor boy, and had few advantages educationally, but he is said to have been "a man of no vices." He did not use tobacco in any form. Had he at the age of ten or eleven or even fifteen become addicted to the use of cigarettes, he would not have reached the President's chair. No cigarette smoker ever has succeeded, or ever will succeed, in reaching the topmost round in the ladder of progress.

Boys, do not be grasshoppers. Look where you expect to land before you jump. If you have high ideals and noble aspirations, have nothing to do with the cigarette. Boys who smoke cigarettes but who are not fiends may sometimes be led to renounce smoking. I talked with two who gave evidence in their lives of the degenerating influence of the smoke. After pointing out the downward career of boys who smoked, I made an appeal to them, and knelt with them in prayer. When we arose, I placed their hands together and asked them to be a help and support to each other, and reminded them that while one could chase a thousand, two could put ten thousand to flight. One year later I was walking along the street of another city when two young men met me and said,

"How do you do, Doctor." I looked at them, and they said, "Do you not remember the two young men you prayed with at such a place?" I answered, "Yes, I remember." "Well, we are the young men. We have not smoked since, and are both here attending school and fitting ourselves to go to a foreign field as missionaries."

While some smokers may be reclaimed, and no case should be regarded as hopeless, yet because it is so difficult to persuade the smoker to see his danger, we should put forth every effort to prevent boys from reaching the border line, or taking even the first step toward it.

### Thoughts for the Thoughtful Lad

TWO of the brightest lads in my medical class are heavy cigarette smokers," said a young man.

"But they are not likely to remain so to the end of the course," remarked his hearer.

"That may be true, for one of them has already begun to fail; but I do not know whether it is his cigarettes or his interest in social activities that is the cause. It may be the latter is partly responsible for his failure; but undoubtedly cigarette smoking must bear the larger share.

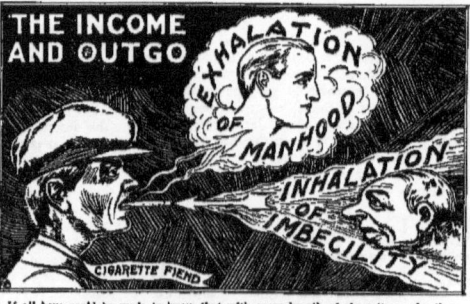

THE INCOME AND OUTGO

EXHALATION OF MANHOOD

INHALATION OF IMBECILITY

CIGARETTE FIEND

If all boys could be made to know that with every breath of cigarette smoke they inhale imbecility and exhale manhood; that they are tapping their arteries as surely and letting their life's blood out as truly as though their veins and arteries were severed; and that the cigarette is a maker of invalids, criminals, and fools, not men,— it ought to deter them some.— Hudson Maxim.

Will you note how these young men stand at graduation time, two years from now? I am sure you will find evidences that tobacco has seriously lessened their efficiency. Observations of this kind have been made many times, and always with the conclusion that smoking injures scholarship."

Said another: "I saw an artist smoking while at his work. He could draw without rule, and with one sweep of his hand, a line across the page as straight as others could with a rule. How could he do this if tobacco is so injurious?"

This artist's natural ability may be so superior that he can have this command of his hand and yet not be at his best. He may not be able to do what he otherwise could have done if he had not subjected his system to the poison. One's own best is what one should give the world. Then again, the poison may be affecting him in a way which will become plainly apparent later in life.

Doubtless this man did not begin smoking until after his brain had been trained to precision. We must never forget that the earlier one begins to smoke the greater the injury wrought by the habit, other circumstances being the same.

### Why You Cannot Smoke

How seriously a moderate use of tobacco may affect you depends upon your age, physical temperament, hereditary tendencies, state of health, work, and home conditions. Even your general knowledge may lend itself to your undoing. Any one of these things may of itself make even a very moderate use of tobacco a serious evil to you, physically, mentally, and spiritually.

Another boy with a less refined ancestry, of a more vigorous hereditary stock, with a different temperament,

(Concluded on page twelve)

# Appendix 2

The interview questionnaire on the following page is unfortunately of poor quality and has not printed very well. So that it can still be included, I have also copied out the text here.

Table 1 - Etiologic Survey

Name...... Age......

1. Have you ever had a lung disease? If so, state time, duration and site of disease:

| | | |
|---|---|---|
| Pneumonia | Asthma | Tuberculosis |
| Bronchiectasis | | |
| Influenza | Lung (unreadable) | Chest injuries |
| Others | | |

2. Do you or did you ever smoke?     Yes          No

3. At what age did you begin to smoke?

4. At what age did you stop smoking?

5. How much tobacco did you average per day during the past 20 years of your smoking?

Cigarettes.........Cigars........Pipes

6. Do you inhale the smoke?          Yes          No

7. Do you have a chronic cough which you attribute to your smoking, especially upon first smoking in the morning? If so, for how long?

Yes          No
Duration

8. Do you smoke before or after breakfast?          Before
After

9. Name the brand or brands, and dates, if any given brand has been smoked exclusively for more than five years.

Changes frequently?
First brand - from 19.... to 19....
Second brand - from 19.... to 19....

10. What kind of jobs have you held? Have you been exposed to dust or fumes while working there? (Use back of page for detailed description of possible exposure)

11. Have you ever been exposed to irritative dusts or fumes outside of your job? In particular have you ever used insecticide spray excessively? If so, state time and duration.

Yes     No     Type....          Duration....

12. How much alcohol do you or have you averaged per day? State time and duration in years.

> Whiskey.... Beer.... Wine....

13. Where were you born and where have you lived most of your life? State the approximate time span you have lived in a certain locality. Up to what grade did you attend school?

> Birthplace.... Home....     Educational Level....

14. State the cause of death of your parents, and of brothers and sisters if any.

15. Size of lesion     Microscopic Diagnosis (Unreadable) Class

> Etiological Class

Interviewer....

TABLE 1.—*Etiologic Survey*

Name:............................................... Age:...............

1. Have you ever had a lung disease? If so, state time, duration and site of disease:

   Pneumonia  Asthma          Tuberculosis      Bronchiectasis
   Influenza  Lung Abscess    Chest Injuries    Others

2. Do you or did you ever smoke?    Yes ☐    No ☐

3. At what age did you begin to smoke?

4. At what age did you stop smoking?

5. How much tobacco did you average per day during the past 20 years of your smoking?

   Cigarettes.............Cigars.............Pipes.............

6. Do you inhale the smoke?    Yes ☐    No ☐

7. Do you have a chronic cough which you attribute to your smoking, especially upon first smoking in the morning? If so, for how long?
   Yes ☐    No ☐
   Duration..........................

8. Do you smoke before or after breakfast?    Before ☐    After ☐

9. Name the brand or brands, and dates, if any given brand has been smoked exclusively for more than five years.

   Change frequently? ☐

First brand—from 19.... to 19....

Second brand—from 19.... to 19....

10. What kind of jobs have you held? Have you been exposed to dust or fumes while working there? (Use back of page for detailed description of possible exposure)

| From | To | Position | Dust or Fumes |
|------|-----|----------|---------------|
|      |     |          |               |
|      |     |          |               |

11. Have you ever been exposed to irritative dusts or fumes outside of your job? In particular have you ever used insecticide spray excessively? If so, state time and duration.
    Yes ☐    No ☐    Type.............Duration.............

12. How much alcohol do you or have you averaged per day? State time and duration in years.
    Whiskey.............Beer.............Wine.............

13. Where were you born and where have you lived most of your life? State the approximate time span you have lived in a certain locality. Up to what grade did you attend school?

    Birthplace.............Home.............Educational Level.............

14. State the cause of death of your parents, and of brothers and sisters if any.

15. *Site of Lesion*          *Microscopic Diagnosis*          *Papanicolaou Class*

    *Etiological Class*

Interviewer ...............................................

278

# Appendix 3

## Membership of the Fair Share for Health Committee

| | |
|---|---|
| *§American Cancer Society, Colorado | †National Jewish Center for Immunology and Respiratory Medicine |
| *§American Lung Association, Colorado | North Colorado Medical Center |
| *AMC Cancer Research Center | Parkview Episcopal Medical Center |
| Avista Hospital | |
| †Boulder County Health Department | Physicians for Social Responsibility |
| Merle C. Chambers | Platte Valley Medical Center |
| *Coalition for a Tobacco-Free Colorado | §Porter Memorial Hospital |
| *Colorado Public Health Association | *Presbyterian-St. Lukes Swedish Health Care System |
| *‡Colorado School Health Council | Rocky Mountain Adventists Healthcare |
| *§Colorado Society for Respiratory Care | *Rocky Mountain Center for Health Promotion and Education |
| †Colorado Tobacco-Free Schools and Communities | Rocky Mountain Oncology Society |
| †§Denver Public Health | Rose Health Care Systems, Inc. |
| *‡Doctors Ought to Care (DOC) | Southern Colorado Clinic |
| †‡El Paso County Health Department | Southern Colorado Health Plan |
| Sam and Nancy Gary | Spalding Rehabilitation Center |

| | |
|---|---|
| *§GASP of Colorado | Sterling Regional Med Center |
| Greeley Medical Center | St. Joseph Hospital |
| Gunnison Valley Hospital | St. Mary-Corwin Hospital |
| Swanee Hunt | Swedish Medical Center |
| International Assoc. for the Study of Lung Cancer | *The Children's Hospital |
| *Jefferson County Dept. of Health and Environment | *University of Colorado Cancer Center |
| *Kaiser Permanente Health Care Program | ‡Weld County Health Department |
| Kate's at 35th Avenue | West Pines Hospital |
| *Larimer County Department of Health | |

†group added to the ASSIST coalition shortly after September 1991
§member of the board of directors of the Coalition for a Tobacco-Free Colorado
‡organization "affiliated with" the Coalition for a Tobacco-Free Colorado

## Appendix 4 - Colorado ASSIST Contractors, 1993-1994

| Organization | Amount |
| --- | --- |
| | |
| American Lung Association of Denver | $60,000 |
| | |
| Arnold Levinson, dba Levinson and Associates | 25,000 |
| | |
| Valley Wide Health Services, Inc. | 25,000 |
| | |
| Larimer County Department of Health and Environment | 35,000 |
| | |
| La Plata County Hospital District | 25,000 |
| | |
| Pueblo City-County Health Department | 35,000 |
| | |
| El Paso County Department of Health and Environment | 45,000 |
| | |
| Boulder County Health Department | 20,000 |
| | |
| Weld County Health Department | 20,000 |
| | |
| Aspen Substance Awareness Project | 15,000 |
| | |

| National Council on Alcohol/Drug Abuse-Mesa County | 15,000 |
|---|---|

Source: Colorado Department of Health ASSIST contractors